Aneurysm Surgery

Published volumes in this series

For Churchill Livingstone
Medical Editor: Miranda Bromage
Copy Editor: Graham Wild
Indexer: Frank Wallis
Design Direction: Erik Bigland
Project Manager: Mark Sanderson
Sales Promotion Executive: Douglas McNaughton

PRACTICE OF SURGERY

Aneurysm Surgery

IRWIN FARIS MB BS (Melb) MD (Monash) FRACS

Professor of Surgery, The University of Melbourne;
Formerly Head, Vascular Surgery Unit,
Royal Adelaide Hospital, Adelaide,
South Australia, Australia

BRIAN BUXTON MB MS (Melb) FRACS

Professor of Cardiac Surgery, Austin Hospital,
Melbourne, Victoria, Australia

WITH CONTRIBUTIONS FROM
FRANCIS QUIGLEY MB MS (Adel) FRACS

Formerly Head, Vascular Surgery Unit, Royal Adelaide Hospital,
Adelaide, South Australia, Australia

GEORGE MATALANIS MB MS (Melb) FRACS

Cardiac Surgeon, Austin Hospital,
Melbourne, Victoria, Australia

LAURENCE DOOLAN FFARCS FANZCA

Director of Operating Room Services, Austin Hospital,
Melbourne, Victoria, Australia

ILLUSTRATIONS BY
PETER COX MMAA

Churchill Livingstone

EDINBURGH HONG KONG LONDON MADRID MELBOURNE NEW YORK AND
TOKYO 1995

CHURCHILL LIVINGSTONE
Medical Division of Longman Group Limited

Distributed in the United States of America by
Churchill Livingstone Inc., 650 Avenue of the
Americas, New York, N.Y. 10011, and by
associated companies, branches and
representatives throughout the world.

First published 1995

ISBN 0 443 04641 7

**British Library Cataloguing in Publication
Data**
A catalogue record for this book is available from
the British Library.

**Library of Congress Cataloging in
Publication Data**
A catalog record for this book is available from
the Library of Congress.

The
publisher's
policy is to use
**paper manufactured
from sustainable forests**

Printed and bound in Great Britain by
William Clowes Limited, Beccles and London

Contents

Contents

Aneurysm surgery presents some of the most varied and challenging experiences encountered by a surgeon. Many of the cases require the routine application of standard techniques and these procedures are carried out daily in major centres. The good results which are obtainable are the result of a number of factors. The most important is careful technique learnt and refined through regular practice by a group of surgeons who regularly discuss their outcomes and clinical problems. Also of major importance are the changes which have occurred in the supportive care given to the patients. This includes the preoperative assessment of coronary artery function, the refinements of intraoperative monitoring and fluid management, and finally the management of respiratory and renal function in the intensive care unit. However, 'Few surgical procedures are fraught with as many possibilities for disastrous complications as that for abdominal aortic aneurysms.' (Imparato 1983). A technical error in dissecting the aorta may result in life-threatening haemorrhage. A carelessly performed anastomosis which results in infection may result in formidable technical difficulties if the limb and life of the patient are to be saved. Secondary operations, as in all surgery, are much more difficult and dangerous than primary operations.

The aim of this book is to illustrate the major procedures performed for arterial aneurysms (excluding those within the cranial cavity). Different surgeons have different techniques and a variety of techniques produce satisfactory outcomes. It is not possible to describe all of these variations but an attempt is made to describe the major alternative methods which are commonly used by experienced surgeons. Emphasis is placed on methods which will minimize the chances of complications because, although it is recognized that complications are inevitable in any branch of surgery, every effort must be made to adopt techniques which will avoid their occurrence. When complications occur, the life of the patient may depend on the ability of the surgical team to rectify the solution as quickly as possible, and techniques for dealing with the major complications are described.

It is hoped that this book will be found useful especially by those who are working with vascular or cardiothoracic surgeons as part of their surgical training and by those not in the full-time practice of vascular surgery who need to operate on patients with aneurysms.

We gratefully acknowledge the work of our collaborators who have made major contributions to the writing of this book. Our colleagues in Adelaide and Melbourne have helped by reading sections of the manuscript and reviewing the drafts of the illustrations.

Geelong and   I.B.F.
Melbourne, 1995   B.F.B.

REFERENCE

Imparato A M 1983 Abdominal aortic surgery: prevention of lower limb
   ischaemia. Surgery 93: 112–116

To Rosemary and Anne, Katherine, Christopher and David

INTRODUCTION AND GENERAL PRINCIPLES

Chapter 1

Introduction

DEFINITION

An aneurysm is a localized dilatation of an artery in which the diameter is increased by at least 50% over that of the expected normal measurement.

This definition requires knowledge of the diameter of the artery and the expected normal diameter. The former is usually easily determined but the latter information is not widely known (see Johnston et al 1991 for details). Detailed guidelines for individual arteries will be discussed in the appropriate sections. Note that the relevant measurement is the external diameter of the vessel. Angiography may underestimate the size of the aneurysm because it will only demonstrate the luminal diameter due to the thrombus which often partly fills the lumen. Guidelines for individual arteries will be discussed in the appropriate sections.

CLASSIFICATION

No single feature allows adequate classification. Factors which are important include the site, aetiology and clinical manifestations.

Site
The site is described anatomically by reference to the artery from which the aneurysm arises. This is important because the natural history varies from site to site. For example, an aneurysm of the common femoral artery may be less dangerous than a smaller aneurysm of the popliteal artery.

Aetiology
Table 1.1 shows a classification of aneurysm according to aetiology. A number of processes which damage or weaken the wall of the artery may cause aneurysm.

The commonest lesions encountered are in elderly patients when the aneurysms

Table 1.1 Aetiology of aneurysm (after Johnston et al 1991)

Congenital, e.g. Ehlers–Danlos, Marfan's
Mechanical, e.g. post-stenotic
    AV fistula-associated
Traumatic
Inflammatory, e.g. Takayasu
    polyarteritis
    periarterial inflammation, e.g. pancreatitis
Infective
Degenerative
    non-specific (atherosclerotic)
Anastomotic

are considered to be *degenerative* in origin. They are commonly labelled 'atherosclerotic' because of the prevalence of atherosclerosis in these patients, and it is said that aneurysm results from weakening the wall by the atherosclerotic process. However, there is reasonable evidence that processes other than atherosclerosis are involved. Patients with aneurysm tend to be older than patients with occlusive diseases. Aneurysmal disease may be part of a diffuse process of arteriomegaly and not associated with stenosing disease.

There are two major forms of *immune vasculitis* which may result in aneurysm formation. Temporal arteritis most commonly affects elderly female patients and predominantly involves the carotid artery and its branches, although any major branch of the aorta may be affected. There have been occasional reports of aneurysm and dissection of the aorta. Takayasu's disease is commonest in young women of east Asian origin and usually presents with occlusion of one or more branches of the aorta. Several patterns of the disease are recognized depending on the distribution of the lesions. Aneurysms occur in about 20% of cases. These may involve the aorta or its major branches.

Infection in an artery rapidly destroys the integrity of the wall and causes aneurysms which rupture. The short time between the appearance of

symptoms and rupture of the aneurysm is characteristic. The commonest cause is infection in a surgical wound which results in disruption of the neighbouring anastomosis. In patients who have not undergone arterial surgery they were formerly associated with bacterial endocarditis but now are most commonly due to intra-arterial injection of non-prescribed drugs. Tuberculosis is seen as a cause of aneurysm in Africa. If acid-fast bacteria are not seen, the histological picture is identical to that described for Takayasu's disease. A non-infective inflammatory process is responsible for the development of the 'inflammatory' aortic aneurysm. These are characterized by a pannus of dense fibrous tissue which varies in extent but which may involve the ureters and may be indistinguishable from the condition of retroperitoneal fibrosis. The aetiology of this process is unknown.

Aneurysm may occur in conditions in which the tunica media of the aorta is weak. The commonest of these conditions is one in which there is generalized dilatation of arteries and is now called *arteriomegaly*. Patients may present with aneurysms at multiple sites, and angiography demonstrates elongated tortuous arteries in which the flow of contrast is very slow. Histological examination of the vessels reveals a reduced number of elastic laminae which presumably allows dilatation to occur. There is a high incidence of thrombotic and embolic complications and increased risks of surgery (Hollier et al 1983). *Marfan's syndrome* is transmitted as an autosomal dominant trait. The exact biochemical deficit is unknown. There is a very high incidence of dilatation of the ascending aorta, aortic valve incompetence, aortic dissection and rupture. A number of varieties of the *Ehlers–Danlos* syndrome have been described. The exact biochemical defect is not known in all cases but in some types which seem particularly prone to arterial problems there is inability to synthesize type III collagen. Many patients with vascular complications have few of the cutaneous and musculoskeletal abnormalities which characterize the syndrome (Hunter et al 1982). Arteries may rupture spontaneously or when punctured, and haemorrhage may be impossible to stop because of the friability of the arterial wall.

The commonest cause of *traumatic aneurysm* is angiography. Blood escapes into the tissues around the artery and is partly contained by laminated thrombus and fibrous tissue. Small lesions may remain stable or resolve but the natural history of larger lesions is to expand and ultimately rupture. The characteristic location for a *poststenotic aneurysm* is distal to the site of compression by a cervical rib. Their development is explained in terms of increased lateral stresses on the arterial wall which follow the blood flow disturbance produced by stenosis. These lesions are dangerous because of the risk of embolism to the arteries of the arm and forearm. *Anastomotic aneurysm* may occur at any site where an anastomosis has been performed. Infection in the anastomosis is the first cause to be considered and a careful search must be made for bacterial pathogens. In some cases infection cannot be demonstrated and it is assumed that local mechanical factors like breaking of a suture or stretching forces on the anastomosis are the cause.

CLINICAL MANIFESTATIONS

These are outlined in Table 1.2. The frequency of the various manifestations varies with the site and the aetiology, e.g. mycotic aneurysms enlarge rapidly and may rupture early in their course wherever they occur.

The complexity of these classifications means that a huge number of combinations are possible. This account will focus on the commoner clinical problems and attempt to enunciate principles which can be applied to other situations.

Table 1.2 Clinical features of aneurysm

None—asymptomatic
Expansion resulting in compression or erosion of surrounding structures
Rupture
Occlusion—local thrombosis or distal embolism
Dissection
Sepsis

REFERENCES

Hollier L H, Stanson A W, Gloviczki P et al 1983 Arteriomegaly: classification and morbid implications of diffuse aneurysmal disease. Surgery 93: 700–708
Johnston K W, Rutherford R B, Tilson M D, Shah D M, Hillier L, Stanley J C 1991 Suggested standards for reporting on arterial aneurysms. Journal of Vascular Surgery 13: 444–450

Chapter 2

Preoperative assessment

Introduction

The improvements in surgical technique and the improvements in supportive care have made aneurysm surgery safer. One consequence of this has been a widening of the indications for surgery so that patients who formerly would not have been offered operation because of the risks of surgery can now be managed safely. The factors which may adversely affect the risks of operation and steps to control these factors are described in this chapter.

INDICATIONS FOR OPERATION

Operation for aneurysm is undertaken to treat complications or, preferably, to prevent their occurrence. The question to be determined is the balance between the risks of operating on a particular patient and the risk of rupture (or other serious complication) if operation is not performed. It is easy to decide to operate on a 60-year-old patient who is shocked because of a ruptured abdominal aortic aneurysm. It is much more difficult to decide in a frail 80-year-old with an asymptomatic abdominal aneurysm.

There are some general principles which help the decision making:

1. Size—larger aneurysms are more likely to rupture.
2. Aetiology—infected false aneurysms are highly likely to rupture in the short term (days).
3. The presence of disseminated malignant disease or advanced cerebrovascular disease contraindicates major surgery.

In many situations the relative risks will need to be assessed, often on the basis of incomplete information.

GENERAL ASSESSMENT OF THE PATIENT

There have been continued improvements in the assessment and management of associated conditions which enable the patient to be made safer for surgery.

Age and sex

It is generally agreed that age alone should not preclude surgery for aneurysm. Demographic data suggest that a man of 80 years has a life expectancy of about 6 years and there is good evidence that surgery can be performed with acceptable mortality (about 10%) in these patients. Certainly it is appropriate to advise surgery in a patient with a large aneurysm who is otherwise fit. In patients with ruptured abdominal aortic aneurysm it is generally agreed that the outlook is worse in patients aged over 80 years. This is largely due to the intolerance of the elderly to hypovolaemia. For reasons which are at present unknown, females with ruptured aneurysm fare worse than male patients.

Risk factors for atherosclerosis

Almost all patients with abdominal aortic aneurysm are current or reformed smokers; hypertension is present in about two-thirds and hypercholesterolaemia in about 50% (DePalma et al 1990). By contrast, diabetes mellitus is less common than in the group presenting with peripheral ischaemia.

Atherosclerotic heart disease

The presence of atherosclerotic heart disease is a major determinant of the prognosis for patients with aneurysm. Thus, when considering the need for surgery, the risks of rupture or other complications of the aneurysm must be balanced against the risks of operation, particularly the risk of perioperative myocardial infarction, which carries a high mortality. Similarly, the major

factor determining long-term survival following successful surgery is the presence of atherosclerotic heart disease.

The detection and management of coronary artery disease is a major focus of the preoperative preparation. A number of studies have attempted to determine the optimal protocols for the evaluation of patients. These have ranged from performing coronary angiography on all patients to a selective approach based on clinical indicators of coronary artery disease.

The high prevalence of coronary artery disease in patients with abdominal aortic aneurysm (up to 66%) is acknowledged; what to do about it remains in dispute. On the one hand, it is argued that coronary artery bypass grafting will protect against perioperative myocardial infarction and late death. On the other hand, it is believed that there is little chance of a significant further reduction in incidence by aggressive surgical therapy of coronary artery disease because modern techniques of management have reduced the incidence of perioperative myocardial infarction to very low levels. Most of the investigations have focused on patients with abdominal aortic aneurysm because of their reported higher prevalence of coronary artery disease. However, there is recent evidence that the incidence of perioperative myocardial infarction may be no less in patients having peripheral vascular procedures and it is arguable that the same protocols should also apply to this latter group.

The algorithm shown in Figure 2.1 is recommended for the assessment of patients with aneurysm. The risk of cardiac complications following surgery is very low in the absence of the defined markers of coronary artery disease. Several methods of screening are available for those with markers of coronary artery disease, and the one chosen will depend on local preferences and experience. Those tested most extensively are the radioisotope tests to estimate either left ventricular ejection fraction or coronary artery perfusion following vasodilator stimulus with dipyridamole. Echocardiography, particularly when performed by the transoesophageal route, is increasingly used as an alternative. Recently, it has been found from continuous ECG monitoring of ambulant patients that ECG changes suggestive of ischaemia occur much more frequently than angina pectoris. It is suggested that patients who exhibit these findings are at greater risk of perioperative myocardial infarction.

Protocols similar to the one described have demonstrated that there is a very low incidence of myocardial infarction in those identified as being at low risk, and this justifies a selective approach to coronary revascularization (Eagle et al 1989).

Respiratory function

Detailed evaluation should be undertaken if there is evidence of severe respiratory disease, typically chronic obstructive airway disease, which is present in one-quarter to one-third of patients. Preoperative preparation should include cessation of smoking for as long as possible, incentive spirometry, treatment of bronchospasm and treatment of bacterial contamination of the lower respiratory tract. Several days may be spent in this preparation.

Renal function

Impaired renal function, indicated by a raised serum creatinine concentration, is present in 20–30% of patients with abdominal aortic aneurysm. Renal function may deteriorate following abdominal aortic surgery. The reasons include hypoperfusion and the effects of aortic clamping (see p. 18), both of which predispose to renal failure.

Patients with pre-existing renal failure should not undergo angiography within 48 hours of planned surgery because of the possible nephrotoxic effect of the contrast medium. The intraoperative measures to maintain renal function are described on page 19.

Haematology

The preoperative assessment should include a history of bleeding disorders and of drugs which might affect the haemostatic processes. The most common drugs encountered are aspirin and other non-steroidal anti-inflammatory agents which suppress the function of the platelets. The skin bleeding time is a useful screening test for these agents. If this is normal, despite the ingestion of aspirin, operation can proceed safely as planned. The prothrombin time and platelet count should also be determined as part of the preoperative evaluation.

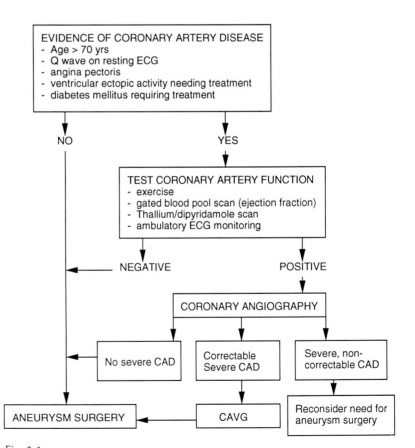

Fig. 2.1
Assessment of coronary artery disease.

Carotid artery stenosis

Routine ultrasound screening of the carotid arteries in patients with aneurysm will demonstrate a significant stenosis of the internal carotid artery in about 10%. If the patient has symptoms appropriate to the carotid lesion, carotid endarterectomy should be performed. The most controversial area is in asymtomatic patients with high-grade stenosis of the internal carotid artery. There is no evidence that the risk of perioperative stroke is increased by these lesions. Many centres would offer these patients an elective procedure on the carotid artery on the basis of evidence which suggests that there is a high incidence of an event (symptoms or occlusion but not necessarily a stroke) from the stenosed artery.

Prevention of infection

Infection of an anastomotic site is a feared complication of arterial surgery. Two important factors which predispose to infection are the insertion of a prosthesis and the performance of surgery in a field contaminated with bacteria. The groin wound is the commonest site of infection. It is heavily contaminated because of its proximity to the anus and because of the presence of lymphatics which may be carrying bacteria draining from infected foci distally in the limb.

There is now good evidence that the incidence of infection is reduced by the use of prophylactic antibiotic therapy. The principles of antibiotic use in these circumstances are that the tissues should contain antibiotic at the time contamination occurs and that antibiotics need not be given for longer than 24 hours after operation. A number of regimens are suitable. Cefotetam 2 g intravenously should be given at the time of induction of anaesthesia. For better cover against staphylococci, flucloxacillin 500 mg should be given with the premedication and 6-hourly for 12–24 hours.

If infection is already present, antibiotic therapy should be directed at the organisms which have been isolated. Particular attention should be paid to the bacteriological techniques used. Special care may be necessary to isolate anaerobic organisms or *Staphylococcus epidermidis*. Discharge of blood or lymph from a wound should be cultured. False aneurysms should be considered to be infected until proven otherwise.

LOCAL ASSESSMENT

Angiography

This remains the cornerstone of vascular investigative techniques, although the newer methods of imaging have expanded the range of available investigations and increased the facility with which they may be applied. In patients with aneurysm, angiography has the major disadvantage that it only shows the lumen of the artery. If there is intraluminal thrombosis present, the diameter of the aneurysm may be seriously underestimated.

Preoperative angiography

This is often essential to provide the surgeon with knowledge of the anatomy of the arterial system adjacent to the lesion to be treated. This allows the surgeon to determine the preferred sites for the anastomoses and plan access accordingly.

The technique which is used most widely is that described by Seldinger. The steps in the procedure are:

1.　The skin is infiltrated with local anaesthetic solution and a small stab wound made at the site for the puncture.
2.　The artery is punctured with a needle.
3.　A guide wire is inserted through the needle to an appropriate position in the arterial tree.
4.　The needle is removed, leaving the guide wire in position.
5.　A catheter is inserted over the guide wire and its tip placed in the required position.
6.　The guide wire is removed.
7.　Contrast is injected through the catheter and appropriate radiographic exposures are made.
8.　The catheter is removed and local pressure applied until the bleeding stops.

In some cases the injection is made directly through the needle, i.e. steps

3–6 are omitted. This technique is suitable when the only images required are of the arterial tree distal to the site of injection. It is the technique used for intraoperative arteriography when the artery may be exposed before puncture.

The image may be obtained by direct exposure of radiographic film. Modern equipment uses digital computer techniques to process the image obtained. This has a number of advantages. The quality of the image obtained is better with a smaller volume of contrast. This may protect the patient against complications, e.g. renal failure, from large doses of contrast. Smaller catheters can be used because smaller volumes of contrast are required and this reduces the chance of injury to the artery. Less radiographic film is required. The disadvantage of the technique is the need for expensive hardware.

Intraoperative angiography
This is an important quality control in vascular surgery. Repeated experience has shown that technical problems in a completed anastomosis of a small artery can be demonstrated in about 10% of operations. Diagnosis of these defects before completion of the operation enables them to be corrected and this reduces the number of reoperations required in the early postoperative period. The smaller the artery being anastomosed, the more critical are minor imperfections of technique.

The usual technique is to puncture the artery above the site to be examined with a 19–21 gauge scalp vein needle and inject contrast. A single exposure can be made after about 10 ml contrast has been injected. If facilities for screening exist, they may allow direct observation of the flow of contrast. A hard copy of a radiograph showing the anastomosis is very valuable. An anastomosis accepted at the end of a long operation may not look so good when submitted to the review of one's

peers. Should late complications, especially graft occlusion, develop, the operative angiogram may provide useful information about the state of the distal arterial tree.

Alternative measures for testing the quality of the repair, including angioscopy and ultrasound examination, may be used instead of angiography. Each anastomosis distal to the bifurcation of the common femoral artery should be checked using one of these methods.

Postoperative angiography
Angiography is no longer needed for the surveillance of arterial reconstructions: computed tomographic (CT) scanning and ultrasound are now the methods of choice. Angiography will usually be required to demonstrate the anatomy of anastomotic false aneurysms prior to their repair (see p. 236) or to determine the patency of the distal arterial tree in cases of graft occlusion.

Ultrasound
This is the area where the most valuable recent advances have occurred. Ultrasound has the major advantage that it is totally non-invasive and free of side-effects. It is thus well tolerated by the patient and can be repeated as necessary. The hardware required is cheaper than that needed for arteriography.

There is continuing development of machines to produce better-quality images. Multiple transducers are used in the examining probe and this produces an image more quickly and of better quality than with earlier machines. The introduction of colour has made the images easier to interpret. Images in the sagittal and coronal planes can be obtained.

It has major applications in patients with aneurysms. These include:

1. Screening asymptomatic patients (see p. 119).
2. Making the diagnosis of aneurysm in symptomatic patients. This applies especially to popliteal and carotid aneurysms, anastomotic aneurysms and aneurysms resulting from radiological trauma in the groin.
3. Evaluating the patency of distal bypass grafts when these are used for the treatment of aneurysm.
4. Treating aneurysms which develop following catheterization of the femoral artery.

Ultrasound is not adequate for the demonstration of the relationship between the neck of an abdominal aortic aneurysm and the renal arteries and, at the present time, only a few centres have extensive experience in diagnosing disease of the visceral vessels.

The method has a high accuracy in the hands of experienced operators, although one of its disadvantages is that clinicians find that the images obtained are more difficult to interpret than the images produced by CT scanning. With earlier equipment the image produced was poorer than that produced by angiography or CT scanning; thus the latter methods have generally been considered necessary preoperatively. However, with the improvement in ultrasound equipment there are a number of situations where operation may be performed using the information provided by ultrasound alone.

Computed tomographic scanning
This technique is also non-invasive (except for the exposure to ionizing radiation) and thus can be repeated without risk to the patient. It has a major application in the assessment of patients with aneurysm. The patient can be examined following the intravenous injection of contrast medium. This allows the differentiation of thrombus in the wall of an aneurysm from the lumen, where the image of the flowing blood

will be shown by the presence of the contrast medium. This ability to demonstrate the wall of the artery is a major advantage over arteriography, in which only the lumen is seen. The two methods provide information which is complementary: CT scanning provides an accurate estimate of the diameter of the aneurysm; arteriography provides information about the arteries above and below the aneurysm.

With newer machines, scanning times are quicker and radiation doses smaller than before. One important limitation to the resolution obtained is that of the thickness of the 'slice' examined. A consequence of this is that the CT scan is often unable to determine precisely the relationship between the neck of an abdominal aortic aneurysm and the renal arteries. This information may be critical in planning surgery.

CT scanning is particularly useful in the assessment of abdominal aortic and iliac aneurysms and in the investigation of possible postoperative complications affecting intra-abdominal grafts.

Magnetic resonance imaging

This method has the advantages that no ionizing radiation or contrast is required and images can be produced in multiple planes. Extensive development work is being undertaken to convert the signals obtained from flowing blood into measurements of blood flow, but this capacity is not yet widely available.

Magnetic resonance (MR) scans can produce excellent images of the blood vessels and their walls. However, there are few situations in vascular surgery where the MR scan provides uniquely valuable information. In patients with aneurysm, it may be of use in complex cases or if complications attributable to

the graft occur postoperatively. It is probably the method of choice for diagnosing aortic dissection, provided the patient's circulation is stable. (It is also the best method for the delineation or the extent of congenital arteriovenous malformations, but these lesions are beyond the scope of this book). The equipment is very expensive and less readily available than the other modalities. The time required to produce an image is long and the image may be degraded by movement of the patient. However, with the improvements in the equipment which are inevitable, MR scans will be performed more frequently in the future.

Details of the use of these investigations are discussed in each section where appropriate. Usually one or the other method provides enough information to plan surgery, but sometimes more than one investigation is needed.

REFERENCES

DePalma R G, Sidawy A N, Giordano J M 1990 In: Greenhalgh R M, Mannick J A, Powell J T (eds) The cause and management of aneurysms. W B Saunders, London, pp 37–46
Eagle K A, Coley C M, Newell J B et al 1989 Combining clinical and thallium data optimizes preoperative assessment of cardiac risk before major vascular surgery. Annals of Internal Medicine 110: 859–866

Chapter 3

Perioperative management

Introduction

The quality of intra- and postoperative care is a major determinant of the outcome in patients with aneurysm. The improvements in this care in recent years have been responsible for the better results obtained and allowed the extension of the indications for surgery to many who would previously have been considered unsuitable because of their age or associated conditions.

TECHNIQUE OF ANAESTHESIA

A variety of techniques for inducing and maintaining anaesthesia may be used. There are advantages and disadvantages for each, so that the choice of technique will depend on the preferences of the anaesthetist and surgeon. The major choice is between major inhalational anaesthesia with or without potent narcotic drugs, and epidural or spinal anaesthesia, with or without a light general anaesthetic. At the present time spinal/epidural anaesthesia is becoming more popular. The advantages include improved cardiac function, better postoperative analgesia and less impairment of pulmonary function. The major disadvantages are the need for increased volume infusion, particularly at the time of removal of the clamps, an increased risk of hypotension in response to haemorrhage, and a small incidence of complications related to the catheter. The major disadvantage of the potent inhalational agents is the cardiac depressant effects.

MONITORING

The minimum requirement for a patient having resection of an aortic aneurysm is for the following functions to be monitored:

1.   Direct arterial pressure
2.   Central venous pressure
3.   ECG
4.   Tissue oxygenation monitored by a pulse oximeter
5.   Urine output monitored by an indwelling urinary catheter

The routine use of the Swan–Ganz catheter is controversial although many centres have adopted this policy. If selective indications are used they include:

1.   Patients with coronary artery disease
2.   Impaired left ventricular function
3.   Elderly (> 75 years)
4.   Patients in whom supracoeliac clamping will be required

Those who use this monitoring as a routine argue for the ability to monitor cardiac output and the unreliability of the central venous pressure as an indicator of left heart filling pressure. Thus problems of low cardiac output and oliguria are easier to manage with a pulmonary artery catheter in place. The disadvantages are the expense of the apparatus and the time necessary for its insertion and monitoring. The decision whether to use these catheters will depend on the preferences of the team in each centre.

Transoesophageal echocardiography has been introduced recently and may prove to be a valuable method of monitoring myocardial ischaemia and left ventricular function during operation.

HAEMODYNAMIC CHANGES

Clamping the aorta has major haemodynamic effects. Variables affecting the magnitude of these changes include the presence of coronary artery disease and the level at which the aorta is clamped, the changes being more pronounced the higher the aorta is clamped. The changes associated with clamping and declamping the infrarenal aorta are shown in Table 3.1. The effect of the raised peripheral resistance is to increase the tension in the ventricular wall. This may lead to subendocardial ischaemia and impaired left ventricular function.

On release of the clamp hypotension, which may cause coronary, renal and cerebral ischaemia, may be lessened by volume loading and reduction in the administration of anaesthetic agents and vasodilator drugs prior to declamping. The surgical technique of gradual declamping is described on page 130. The effects of declamping are also more pronounced the higher the clamp is applied.

Table 3.1   Haemodynamic effects of application and removal of aortic clamp

Measurement	Clamping		Declamping	
Cardiac output	Decrease	20–30%	Increase	0–15%
Mean arterial pressure	Increase	10%	Decrease	5–35%
Heart rate	No change		Increase	
Systemic vascular resistance	Increase	33%	Decrease	10–30%
Stroke volume	Decrease	15–20%	Increase	0–10%
Filling pressures	Variable		Decrease	0–30%

MAINTENANCE OF CARDIAC FUNCTION

In patients with impaired cardiac function the perioperative management may include preoperative volume loading to determine the left atrial pressure which produces maximum cardiac output. This may be performed the day prior to surgery (Grindlinger et al 1980) and requires the insertion of a Swan–Ganz catheter. Myocardial ischaemia during operation may occur at any time but is particularly likely on application and removal of the aortic clamp. The risk is increased the higher the clamp is applied. Perioperative use of beta-blocking agents may reduce the incidence of perioperative myocardial infarction.

During operation a number of steps may be taken to assist the maintenance of cardiac function:

1. Monitoring cardiac output by thermal dilution using the Swan–Ganz catheter and maintaining fluid balance, particularly filling pressure, for optimal cardiac output ($> 2\,l/min/m^2$).
2. Before the aorta is clamped, an infusion of sodium nitroprusside ($5-150\,\mu g/min$) or nitroglycerine ($0.25-1\,\mu g/kg/minute$) may be commenced. The dose required to control the blood pressure after application of the clamp is variable. The reduction in cardiac afterload will improve coronary perfusion while maintaining systemic arterial pressure at acceptable levels. The efficacy of these infusions in preventing myocardial ischaemia and infarction has not been proven conclusively.
3. If blood pressure remains low despite adequate filling pressure, inotropic support for the myocardium is required. Dopamine ($5-500\,\mu g/min$) may be used.
4. In rare cases intra-aortic balloon counterpulsation may be necessary.

FLUID MANAGEMENT

It is assumed that the patient comes to the operation with an adequate circulating blood volume (for discussion regarding fluid loading see above). Many anaesthetists choose fluid replacement regimens which result in a modest reduction in haematocrit (although myocardial oxygenation will be impaired by too great a reduction). Crystalloid solution will be required to replace third-space losses. The volume required will be greater in patients having spinal/epidural anaesthesia.

PRESERVATION OF RENAL FUNCTION

Aortic clamping results in a reduction in renal blood flow and an increase in renal vascular resistance. Both these changes predispose to renal failure. The effects can be reduced by careful attention to fluid replacement. Maintenance of optimal cardiac function will help maintain renal blood flow and thus renal function. In most patients, the administration of mannitol is unnecessary. In patients with pre-existing elevated serum creatinine, renal failure is more common. Adequate hydration is essential and a Swan–Ganz catheter may assist in maintaining this state. During operation, these patients should receive $12.5-25\,g$ mannitol intravenously and great care must be taken to avoid renal ischaemia. If supracoeliac clamping is required, mannitol should be administered prior to release of the aortic clamp.

Postoperative oliguria should be treated by $400-500\,ml$ boluses of saline. Diuretics which are tubular poisons (such as frusemide) should only be given if there is unequivocal evidence that the circulation is adequately filled.

RESPIRATORY MANAGEMENT

There is some evidence that epidural anaesthesia may lessen the postoperative impairment of respiratory function. In most patients the endotracheal tube is not removed until the patient has been settled in the intensive care unit. The duration of ventilation required depends on many factors, including the preoperative condition of the patient, the presence of chronic obstructive airways disease, the length of the procedure and the amount of blood infused. Before extubation, the patient should be normothermic, haemodynamically stable, awake, and demonstrate adequate ventilation and gas exchange without mechanical assistance. If there are concerns about peripheral ischaemia or continuing bleeding, ventilation should be continued.

BLOOD REPLACEMENT

The amount of blood required is one of the major predictors of outcome following surgery for abdominal aortic aneurysm; increased transfusion is associated with myocardial infarction, respiratory and renal failure, and death. The average requirement for blood replacement is said to be 2 litres for elective resection of an abdominal aortic aneurysm and double that amount if the aneurysm is ruptured. In a number of patients elective resection can be performed without homologous blood transfusion. Blood loss is greatest in patients with thoracoabdominal aneurysm.

In recent years methods of autotransfusion have been introduced to reduce the need for transfusion of homologous blood. Use of autologous blood eliminates the possibility, variable as it is, of transmission of infection and of transfusion reactions. A number of techniques are available:

1. Preoperative donation. Many centres have protocols for the collection of blood prior to elective surgery. This commonly involves donation of one unit each week for 2 or 3 weeks, the last donation being not less than 10 days before planned surgery. This can be simply and cheaply organized and has the potential for considerable savings in the requirement for homologous blood. However, it may be difficult to implement these programmes because of administrative and social factors. Many patients require operation too soon to allow collection of blood.

Up to 1 litre of blood may be collected in the immediate pre-anaesthetic period for infusion during the operation. The circulating volume is maintained by the infusion of a similar volume of crystalloid or colloid. Those who believe in the haemodynamic advantages produced by haemodilution

will favour using this method. A similar result can be obtained by replacing the first litre of blood lost during the procedure with crystalloid solution.

2. Intraoperative autotransfusion. It is in this area that the greatest advances have occurred. Several methods are available.

A simple container attached to the suction line may be used to trap and filter the blood. When the container is full, it is disconnected and passed to the anaesthetist for infusion. The patient must be heparinized. In general the blood cannot be replaced quickly enough to avoid homologous transfusion.

With the more elaborate devices the blood is washed and filtered to remove aggregates before adding it to a container from which it can be reinfused. These devices are more expensive and may need a dedicated operator. The components of the systems (Fig. 3.1) include:

a. A double-lumen suction tube which collects the blood at low pressure suction to avoid damage to the red blood cells. Through the second lumen anticoagulant is added to the region of the tip of the sucker.
b. A reservoir from which blood is added to.
c. A centrifuge in which the blood is washed. The supernatant is discarded.
d. The washed red blood cells are stored in a reinfusion bag. The haematocrit of the infused blood is 50–60%.

The cost of consumable components is similar to the cost of about two units of homologous blood. Recent developments have produced machines which are capable of preparing the blood more rapidly with less damage to its components.

There are several possible adverse effects of autotransfusion. These include:

a. Damage to the erythrocytes. There is a rise in the level of plasma-free haemoglobin but this is usually of no consequence. The survival of the transfused cells is similar to that of homologous blood.
b. Loss of coagulation factors. The concentrations of fibrinogen and factors V and VIII are higher than in banked blood. Platelets are removed from the blood during processing.
c. Transmission of bacteria is possible with this technique, so that it should only be used in clean operating fields.

CLOTTING FACTORS

Administration of clotting factors is seldom necessary in elective surgery of abdominal aortic aneurysm. However, in thoracic and thoracoabdominal aneurysm clotting factors may be given as a routine, e.g. fresh frozen plasma after each 2–3 units of blood and 10–16 packs of fresh platelets when blood is restored to the graft (Crawford 1990). If whole blood is used for transfusion, there is a reduced requirement for platelets and clotting factors. In patients with ruptured aneurysm, fresh frozen plasma and 6–8 packs of platelets should be given after blood transfusion of 4–5 litres of blood. It is preferable to administer these products in order to prevent development of coagulopathy than to try to control bleeding once a coagulopathy has become established. The use of the thromboelastograph to guide therapy is described on page 43.

CONTROL OF BODY TEMPERATURE

Large-volume infusions of cold fluid and prolonged exposure of the abdominal viscera make patients undergoing surgery for aneurysm particularly liable to hypothermia. Routine measures should be taken to reduce this risk. These include warming of inspired air and infused fluid, and a heating blanket on the operating table (cf. p. 40).

POSTOPERATIVE CARE

Careful monitoring of haemodynamic variables during the early postoperative period is essential to minimize the chances of myocardial infarction or renal failure.

Most patients will be transferred to the intensive care unit, receiving mechanical ventilation via the endotracheal tube. Meticulous toilet of the airway and aggressive chest physiotherapy should be routine measures.

Postoperative analgesia is an important consideration. This may be assisted by epidural administration of analgesics or one of the modern techniques of pain control such as patient-controlled analgesia.

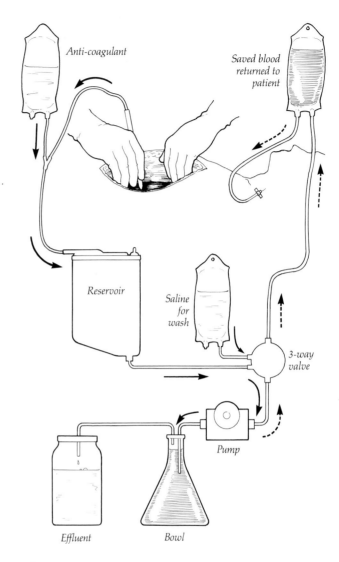

Fig. 3.1
Diagram of red blood cell scavenger.

REFERENCES

Crawford E S 1990 Thoraco-abdominal and proximal aortic replacement for extensive aortic aneurysmal disease. In: Greenhalgh R M, Mannick J A, Powell J T (eds) The cause and management of aneurysms. W B Saunders, London, pp 351–372
Grindlinger G A, Vegas A M, Manny J, Bush H L, Mannick J A, Hechtman H B 1980 Volume loading and vasodilators in abdominal aortic aneurysmectomy. American Journal of Surgery 139: 480–486

Chapter 4

General techniques

PRINCIPLES OF OPERATIONS

The basic steps in any vascular surgery procedure can be defined as:

1. Exposure
2. Control
3. Heparinization
4. Application of clamps
5. Direct arterial procedures

There are a number of components which may or may not be used in particular circumstances:

a. No repair may be performed, e.g. Hunterian ligation for popliteal aneurysm.
b. The distal circulation may be restored by a number of methods:

 i. Interposition graft, usually placed within the bed of an aneurysm
 ii. Bypass graft
 iii. Direct repair, e.g. of aortocaval fistula

c. Excision of the aneurysm may or may not be undertaken.

6. Release of clamps and achieving haemostasis
7. Checking distal circulation
8. Closure of wounds

Exposure

It is an essential requirement in vascular surgery that the blood vessels to be dissected must be adequately displayed. In general, vessels are approached by the most direct route and the whole of the vessel displayed. This means that exposure takes precedence over the cosmetic appearance of the scar. Exceptions to this rule include incisions on the flexor aspect of joints, e.g. the posterior approach to the popliteal artery (see p. 221). Tissues are generally incised as widely as necessary. Thus the clavicle may be divided to expose the junction between the subclavian and axillary arteries. However, the inguinal ligament is usually preserved in the exposure of the distal external iliac artery and proximal common femoral artery. The medial head of the gastrocnemius muscle and the tendons of sartorius, gracilis and semitendinosus muscles may be preserved during the medial approach to the popliteal artery. It should be noted that, in both situations, the muscles and tendons may be divided if necessary to obtain optimum exposure.

Control

This term means being able to occlude all arteries in the field of the procedure, so that when the artery is opened there is no continuing leakage of blood into the operative field. The vessels dissected include the proximal 'inflow' artery, the distal 'outflow' vessels and all significant branches arising in the field of the operation. The outflow vessels may include major branches of the inflow artery (e.g. the superficial femoral and profunda femoris arteries) and, in cases of arteriovenous communication, the draining veins.

There are two cardinal rules in dissecting an artery. They are:

1. The safest plane is found as close as possible to the wall of the artery.
2. It is dangerous to attempt to pass an instrument blindly around an artery.

In normal arteries there is adjacent to the artery a plane which is easily found and which comprises fine strands of connective tissue which are easily divided. This dissection is carried out with scissors and forceps. Care must be taken not to damage the artery by grasping it with forceps. The soft tissues are grasped away from the artery (Fig. 4.1) and stretched. Some of the dissection can be carried out by pushing the artery with the closed scissors (Fig. 4.2) or by inserting the tip of a finger and using it gently to break down the connective tissue. In displaying an artery which has been dissected at a previous operation, exposure may be much more difficult because of the obliteration of the plane of dissection. In these circumstances the dissection is carried out with toothed forceps (e.g. Adson's) and scalpel (with a number 15 blade). This dissection may be tedious and dangerous, but less damage is likely to occur from a small clean cut to a vessel than from the tearing that is produced by attempting to establish a plane by opening scissors in a confined space.

The dissection continues until the artery can be encircled, when a tape is placed around the artery by inserting the end of the tape in the tip of forceps placed behind the artery (Fig. 4.3). Tapes 2–4 mm wide are placed around vessels which will be clamped. The tape acts as a safeguard against inadvertent removal of the clamp during the procedure and allows control of haemorrhage should excessive bleeding from the anastomosis occur on release of the clamp. Smaller arteries may be controlled by passing a silk ligature twice around them. These ligatures when pulled tight will occlude the vessel. The ligature is removed by dividing one thread as close as possible to the vessel it surrounds and pulling gently on the other thread. In some situations it is safer to control vessels without completely encircling them. These situations include the common iliac arteries (and sometimes the aorta) in patients with abdominal aortic aneurysm and the profunda femoris artery in cases of anastomotic false aneurysm (see text for details).

Heparinization

Stagnation of blood is one of the factors which predisposes to thrombosis. Blood flow in the arterial tree distal to the clamps is much reduced and, especially if it is in contact with ulcerated atheromatous plaques, may clot. This causes distal ischaemia after blood flow is restored. Heparin is given to prevent this distal thrombosis. Not all surgeons agree that heparin is necessary and there are some situations, e.g. ruptured abdominal aortic aneurysm, where many surgeons would not give heparin. However, heparin is administered in most arterial operations although it is conceded that frequently dose and control of effect are not closely monitored.

Heparin may be given by the intravenous administration of 1 mg/kg, 2–3 minutes before the clamps are applied. Some surgeons give an empirical dose of 5000 or 10 000 units (50 or 100 mg). Most vascular procedures are complete within 1 hour of clamping, but more heparin should be given if the clamps are applied for longer. The usual regimen is to give half the original dose hourly following the first dose until circulation is restored.

If haemostasis is good, it is not necessary to reverse the heparin at the end of the procedure. However, if reversal is indicated to aid haemostasis, protamine 25 mg is given intravenously. This drug must be given slowly because it has a direct depressant effect on the myocardium.

An alternative method of heparin administration is to give it regionally rather than systemically. This has the advantage of not interfering with haemostasis at the suture line. Heparin is given through a cannula inserted into a distal artery. Heparin 2000 units is mixed with 100 ml saline. About 20 ml of this solution is injected into the distal vessels (into each common iliac artery if the aorta is clamped). This may be repeated at hourly intervals if necessary.

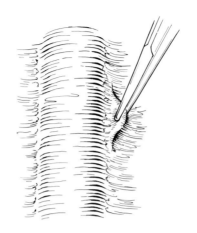

Fig. 4.1
Plane of dissection close to artery.

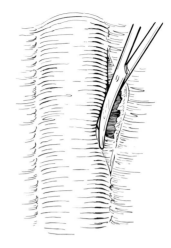

Fig. 4.2
Separation of tissues using closed scissors.

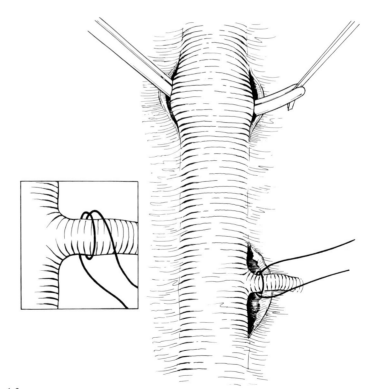

Fig. 4.3
Encircling artery with tape; controlling small branch with ligature. Inset: detail of placement of ligature.

Application of clamps

Clamps suitable to the diameter and thickness of the artery are applied at the sites at which tapes have been placed. This is discussed in more detail in the appropriate sections.

The artery is opened after incising with a scalpel (a pointed number 11 blade is commonly used) and the incision enlarged with scissors. If all the blood vessels entering and leaving the segment have been occluded there will be no bleeding. There are many situations in aneurysm surgery where this ideal is not attainable. Two examples are bleeding from lumbar arteries when an abdominal aortic aneurysm is opened and bleeding from the profunda femoris artery in cases of anastomotic aneurysm of the femoral artery. Techniques for dealing with this bleeding are described in the appropriate sections.

Direct arterial procedures

In aneurysm surgery the commonest techniques used for reconstruction are interposition and bypass grafting. In rare circumstances (e.g. false aneurysm of the common femoral artery following coronary angiography) it may be possible to perform a direct repair of the artery. Sometimes (e.g. in aortobi-iliac grafting for aorto-iliac aneurysm) the procedure is a combination of interposition and bypass.

Suturing technique

There are two properties of a good arterial anastomosis. They are that it is patent and not bleeding. How best to achieve these outcomes requires the use of a variety of suturing techniques depending on the artery being sutured. There are two important general principles when suturing arteries. These are, first, that the artery wall is handled as little as possible. Grasping the artery wall with forceps may result in fracturing of atheromatous plaques and subsequent tearing out of the sutures.

Second, it is better to place the suture into the luminal side of the artery. This tends to secure rather than raise plaques and flaps which may either weaken the wall or narrow the anastomosis. In large arteries like the aorta deep sutures may be placed 2–3 mm apart (see Fig. 8.14). In small arteries, very fine sutures, 1 mm or less apart, may be used.

Interposition grafting

This involves end-to-end anastomoses between the graft and the artery. The wall of the aneurysm may be excised or the graft may be placed in the lumen of the aneurysm. Placement of a straight tube graft for repair of an abdominal aortic aneurysm (see p. 124) is the commonest example of this method. The technique of end-to-end anastomosis is illustrated. If the arteries are sufficiently mobile to allow them to be rotated, the technique illustrated in Figures 4.4 and 4.5 is used. Single-ended sutures (labelled A and B in the figures) are placed at each side of the anastomosis and tied. The short ends of the sutures (labelled A2 and B2) are held in mosquito forceps. Suturing starts at one side of the anastomosis (with suture A1) and progresses towards the suture at the other side (B1 in Fig 4.4). When this section is complete the suture A is tied to the short end of suture B. The ends of the vessels are rotated so that the unsutured part of the anastomosis is towards the operator. This is accomplished by passing needles A1 and B1 and the short end of suture B (B2) behind the vessels to the opposite side. The short end of suture A is moved across the anterior aspect of the vessels to the side opposite from which it originated. The suturing continues with suture B from the original starting side until the anastomosis is complete (Fig. 4.5).

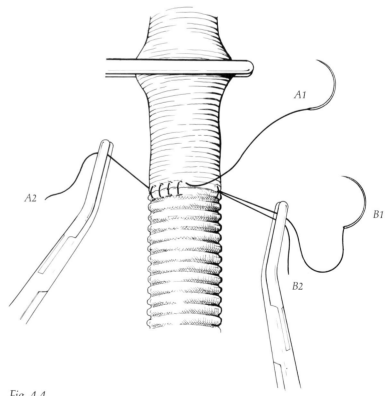

Fig. 4.4
End-to-end anastomosis: anterior suture line.

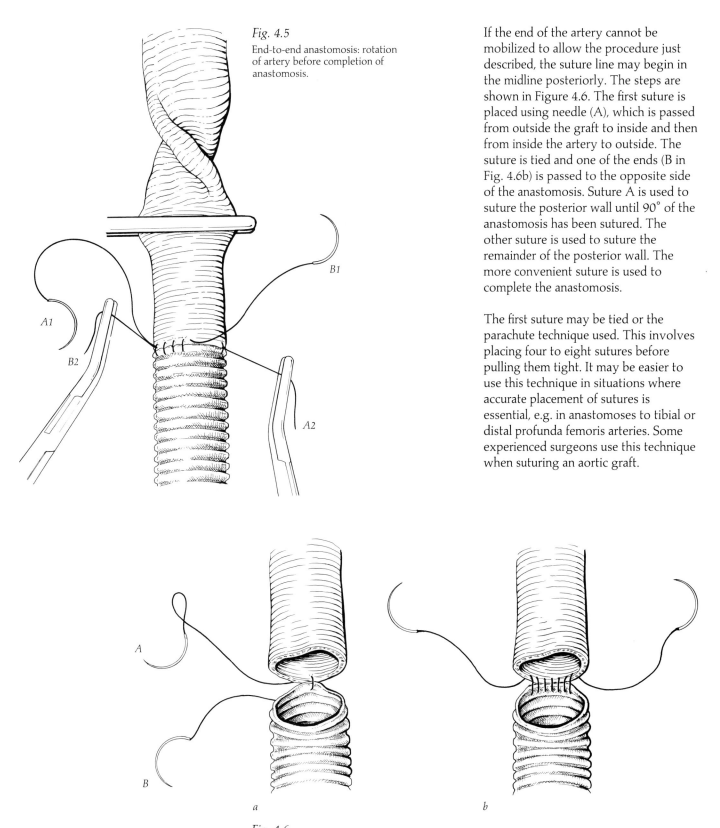

Fig. 4.5

End-to-end anastomosis: rotation of artery before completion of anastomosis.

If the end of the artery cannot be mobilized to allow the procedure just described, the suture line may begin in the midline posteriorly. The steps are shown in Figure 4.6. The first suture is placed using needle (A), which is passed from outside the graft to inside and then from inside the artery to outside. The suture is tied and one of the ends (B in Fig. 4.6b) is passed to the opposite side of the anastomosis. Suture A is used to suture the posterior wall until 90° of the anastomosis has been sutured. The other suture is used to suture the remainder of the posterior wall. The more convenient suture is used to complete the anastomosis.

The first suture may be tied or the parachute technique used. This involves placing four to eight sutures before pulling them tight. It may be easier to use this technique in situations where accurate placement of sutures is essential, e.g. in anastomoses to tibial or distal profunda femoris arteries. Some experienced surgeons use this technique when suturing an aortic graft.

Fig. 4.6

(a) End-to end anastomosis: placement of first suture. (b) Posterior wall sutured from within artery.

Bypass grafting

In these procedures the arteries entering and leaving the aneurysm are occluded and a bypass graft placed to restore blood flow. A common example of this is the treatment of popliteal aneurysm, when a bypass graft is placed between the superficial femoral artery above the aneurysm and the popliteal artery below.

The anastomoses are usually fashioned between the end of the graft and the side of the artery. An ellipse may be removed from the wall of the artery but this is not necessary. The technique of suturing is as shown in Figure 4.7a–c. It is customary to begin suturing at the acute angle between the graft and artery, which is called the heel of the anastomosis. The first suture using needle A is placed from outside the graft into its lumen and then from inside the artery to the outside. The sutures are tied and one of the needles (B in Fig. 4.7b) is passed beneath the graft to the side away from the operator. Suturing is shown proceeding with needle A. When the first side of the anastomosis is about half complete, any redundant corner of graft is excised as shown in Figure 4.7b. Trimming is best carried out at this time because the graft is firmly held by the sutures which have been placed and judgement of the correct length is easiest. Figure 4.7c shows how needle B has been used to suture the side away from the operator to the apex of the anastomosis. This is the area where narrowing of the anastomosis is tolerated least. Suturing should continue with needle B until needle A is reached, when the flushing procedure described below is undertaken and the sutures tied.

The parachute technique may be used as shown in Figure 4.8. In this case suturing has begun at the apex of the anastomosis using needle A. This method has the advantage that it allows easier vision of the critical apex region.

The next sutures would be placed using needle B passed first back into the lumen of the graft, then into the luminal surface of the artery. Two or three sutures would be placed in this way before the threads are pulled tight.

Release clamps

When the anastomosis is about 75–80% complete, it should be flushed to remove loose thrombus and other debris from the lumen. This is not so important for the proximal anastomosis because the graft can be flushed during the performance of the distal anastomosis. However, if desired, the proximal anastomosis can be flushed by loosening the proximal clamp for one or two heart beats. The blood is sucked from the field, which is then irrigated with the heparinized saline solution (5000 units heparin in 200 ml saline). Removal of debris from the distal circulation is critical. A suitable routine is as follows:

1. Loosen the proximal clamp as described.
2. Remove the blood by suction.
3. Release the distal clamp and check for back-bleeding from the distal circulation.
4. Remove this blood by suction.
5. Liberally irrigate the lumen in the area of the anastomosis with heparinized saline solution.
6. Complete the suture line.
7. Release the proximal clamp first to allow entrapped air to escape through the suture line.
8. If there are two distal clamps, remove the clamp from the less critical vessel first; e.g. the clamp is removed from the internal iliac before the external iliac artery and from the external carotid artery before the internal carotid. This will allow any thrombus or other debris to be carried by the blood flow into the less critical territory.

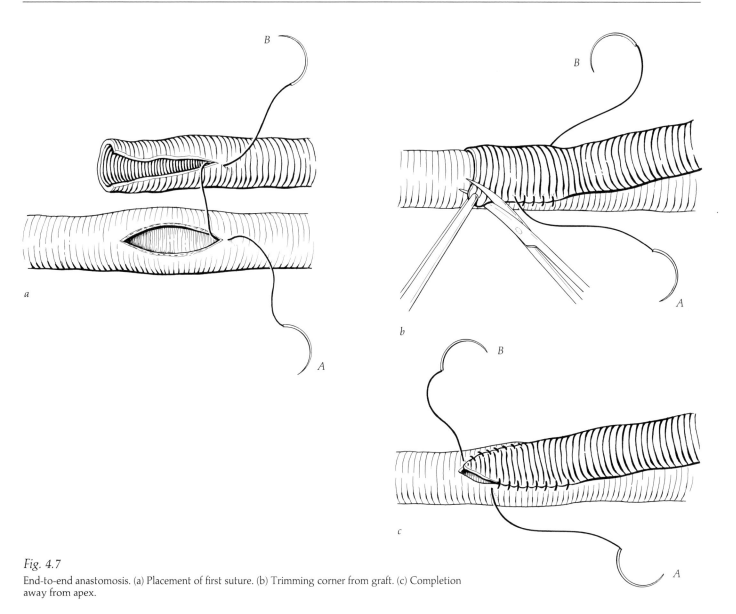

Fig. 4.7
End-to-end anastomosis. (a) Placement of first suture. (b) Trimming corner from graft. (c) Completion away from apex.

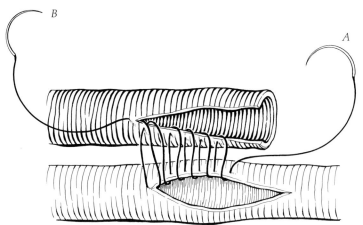

Fig. 4.8
Parachute technique.

Achieve haemostasis

In almost all anastomoses there is bleeding from the suture line. A dry gauze square is placed over the suture line and pressure applied for 5 minutes. Removal of the gauze will usually show that the suture line is dry.

If bleeding persists, the steps to be taken depend on the nature and severity of the bleeding. Continued bleeding from very small holes may be controlled by the application of haemostatic gauze, pressure as described above and waiting a further 5 minutes. If bleeding continues the heparin activity should be reversed (see p. 25). The need for further sutures may be a matter requiring fine judgement. Placement of additional sutures may cause further bleeding.

Leaks where the blood comes out in a continuous spurt require attention. If there are significant leaks the proximal clamp is reapplied. *Additional sutures are never tied unless the inflow is controlled.* Attempts to do so will result in tearing of the arterial wall and worse bleeding. Remember that it is not necessary to tie these sutures too tightly. The tension in the wall when flow is restored will tend to tighten the suture and may produce tearing if the suture is too tight.

The major causes of leaks from a vascular suture line and their treatment are:

1. Sutures too far apart. Place a single suture if the leak is small or (more commonly) a cross-stitch.
2. Sutures too loose (Fig. 4.9).

a. Tighten the loose sutures by placing a nerve (sympathectomy) hook under the loose suture(s) until a single loop is produced.
b. Pass a suture (labelled X in the figure) through this loop and secure the ends of the suture with a haemostatic forcep.

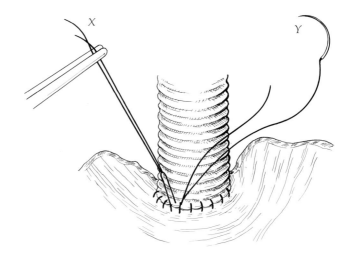

Fig. 4.9
Technique for dealing with loose sutures.

c. Place a single suture (labelled Y) through the graft and artery wall close to the loop and tie the suture.
d. Tie one end of the last-placed suture (Y) to the loop, using the suture through the loop (X) to ensure that the loop is incorporated in the knot.
e. Remove suture X.
f. Cut the ends of the remaining suture.

3. Sutures tearing out. If a single suture has partially torn the wall it can be treated with a cross-stitch as shown in Figure 4.10. A significant split in the wall of the artery may occur during the performance of the anastomosis. It is treated by placing a mattress suture at the sides of the apex of the split as shown in Figure 4.11. Note that the sutures are placed on either side of the apex of the tear. If a suture is placed deep to the apex, a much larger split will result if, as is likely, this last suture also tears out.
4. Bleeding from suture holes in graft. This is worst with polytetrafluoroethylene (PTFE) grafts. Holes are controlled by packing (with or without haemostatic gauze) and patience. Reversal of the heparin may be necessary if the bleeding is continuing when both anastomoses are complete.

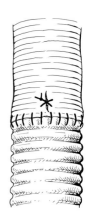

Fig. 4.10
Split after completion of suture line.

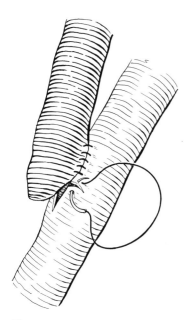

Fig. 4.11
Split sutured during anastomosis.

Check distal circulation

Some objective assessment of the distal circulation is necessary after every arterial procedure. This may range from palpation of the femoral pulses following repair of an abdominal aortic aneurysm to intraoperative angiography or ultrasonography when the distal anastomosis is to an artery smaller than the common femoral artery. The technique of intraoperative angiography, which is the method most widely used, has been described on page 13.

If the distal arterial tree is unobstructed, the ankle pulses should return after restoration of the circulation and distal pressures should be normal. If there are distal obstructions, pulses may not be felt but the colour of the skin should return to normal and the temperature gradient between warm and cool should progressively move distally during the succeeding 24 hours. Similarly, the ankle pressure index (the ratio of ankle to arm systolic blood pressure) may not return to its normal level of > 0.9 but it should be at least as high as it was preoperatively and increase over the first 1–2 days postoperatively.

Close wounds

Closure of the wounds must be performed carefully. Abdominal aortic aneurysm was one of the conditions recognized as being at high risk of abdominal wound dehiscence. The use of mass closure techniques has virtually eliminated this complication. In areas where the skin may be ischaemic, it must be handled very gently. Wound necrosis may complicate femorodistal bypass surgery in up to 30% of cases. In these areas the skin must not be grasped with heavy forceps. Fine-toothed forceps (e.g. Adson's) are suitable.

A drain may be placed if there is a risk of continuing drainage of blood or lymph. However, a drain will not prevent a haematoma from forming if haemostasis at the anastomosis has been inadequate. Drains are not necessary adjacent to an aortic anastomosis but many surgeons place drain tubes adjacent to femoral, popliteal and carotid suture lines, although there is no strong evidence that they are essential. These drains may be removed on the morning following operation.

GRAFTS AND SUTURES

Grafts

The placement of prosthetic grafts down to and including the level of the common femoral artery has proved to be a remarkably durable procedure despite the fact that formation of an endothelial lining does not occur further than 1 cm or so from the anastomosis. Various techniques of manufacture have been used (see Table 126). The major variations have been in the porosity of the graft. Increased porosity allows easier ingrowth of fibrous tissue but allows leakage of blood at the time of operation. Less porous grafts are stiffer and harder to handle and suture. The latest development has been to fill the interstices of a porous (knitted) graft with gelatine or albumin. Grafts impregnated during manufacture are widely available but a technique for albumin impregnation is described on page 58. These grafts are softer than woven grafts and do not leak blood. Enzymatic digestion of the gelatine or albumin allows the ingrowth of fibrous tissue. Grafts made from expanded PTFE do not leak blood through the interstices and are able to be incorporated by the ingrowth of fibrous tissue. Their disadvantages are that until recently they have been inelastic, so that judgement of length is critical; also there is a tendency for leakage from suture holes to occur, and this may produce bleeding which is annoyingly difficult to control.

There is no proven difference in patency or complication rate between any of these grafts used within the abdomen or chest.

In the limbs, autologous vein is the graft of choice. The preferred donor site is the ipsilateral long saphenous vein. If this is not available, the contralateral long saphenous vein, either short saphenous vein or a suitable arm vein may be used. The patency of prosthetic grafts is clearly inferior to vein grafts in the lower limb. Synthetic grafts may be used in cases where there is no suitable vein or during urgent surgery on frail patients when the operating time can be reduced by using a prosthesis. Specific examples illustrating these principles are given in the text.

Sutures

Monofilament sutures have replaced braided sutures in most situations. Polypropylene or similar polymer is the material most commonly used. Sutures made from PTFE may be used when that material is being used as the prosthesis. These sutures reduce the amount of bleeding from the suture line with this graft material. The calibre of the material used varies with the site, e.g.

3/0 Aorta, common iliac artery
4/0 External iliac artery, common femoral artery
5/0 Common femoral artery, profunda femoris artery, popliteal artery
6/0 Internal carotid artery, tibial arteries

In repair of thoracic aneurysm there are two significant variations in the materials used. When a new valve or valved conduit is being inserted (see p. 58) interrupted braided sutures may be used. The second variation is the more frequent use of pledgets of Teflon to reinforce the suture line and to prevent the sutures from tearing out. This technique may be used to reinforce a difficult anastomosis in the abdominal aorta.

THORACIC AND THORACOABDOMINAL ANEURYSM

Chapter 5

Principles of repair of thoracic aortic aneurysms

George Matalanis   **Laurence Doolan**   **Brian Buxton**

Introduction

In considering the surgical approach to aneurysms of the thoracic aorta, careful selection of patients is essential. For asymptomatic patients, the risks of surgery are weighed against the knowledge of the natural history of the underlying condition. For patients who present acutely, such as those with ruptured or leaking aneurysms, stringent selection criteria may be relaxed. Planning a thoracic aortic resection is vital. The type of surgical procedure is determined by the aetiology of the underlying condition, the site, size and shape of the aneurysm, and the organ preservation required.

CLINICAL PRESENTATION

Aneurysms may be found incidentally on routine chest X-rays or computed tomography (CT) scans, or during investigation of chronic chest or upper back pain, aortic regurgitation murmur, spontaneous onset of hoarseness which, in the presence of an aneurysm, may be due to recurrent laryngeal nerve palsy, or digital ischaemia (the 'blue toe syndrome') which may be due to microthromboemboli.

Patients may present acutely with sudden severe chest or upper back pain associated with collapse and hypotension secondary to acute dissection, leakage or rupture of an aneurysm. Traumatic rupture of the aorta from sudden deceleration injury may be suspected when the mediastinum is widened on a chest X-ray. Acute dissection may cause severe aortic regurgitation, coronary, arch vessel, visceral, spinal or iliofemoral artery obstruction. Acute myocardial infarction, transient ischaemic attack or stroke, paraplegia, gut infarction or limb ischaemia may be the result of thromboembolism. Mycotic aneurysms often present with septicaemia, while haemoptysis and haematemesis may herald the arrival of massive exsanguinating haemorrhage from aorto-oesophageal, aortobronchial or aortotracheal fistula.

Assessment
The goal of preoperative investigations is twofold: firstly, to provide a detailed assessment of the pathology present; and secondly, to give an overall assessment of the patient's general fitness. Angiography, CT and magnetic resonance imaging (MRI) scanning, and echocardiography are all very useful tools to define the nature and extent of aortic pathology, the diameter of the various segments of the aorta and the presence of complications. CT scanning can accurately assess the size of aortic

aneurysms, define the presence of dissection, local complications such as intraluminal thrombus and leakage, renal size and perfusion. However, CT scanning gives limited information about the aortic branches. Angiography, on the other hand, gives very accurate details of the aortic branches and their relationship to disease processes. Angiographic assessment of aortic diameter can be erroneous in the presence of intraluminal thrombus (Barbetseas 1992, Chan 1991). Echocardiography (Erbel et al 1989) and in particular transoesophageal echocardiography can image the thoracic aorta very well and in addition provide valuable information regarding myocardial contractility and heart valve function. Echocardiography unfortunately cannot provide information below the diaphragm. MRI scanning (Nienaber et al 1992) gives similar information to CT scanning, with the added benefit of coronal and oblique reconstructions. Unfortunately, the expense, long examination time and restriction to major centres make it a less widely applicable investigation.

In an emergency, rapid assessment of the aortic pathology is required so that definitive surgical repair can be expedited. Transoesophageal echocardiography is ideally suited for this. The procedure can be performed and results obtained within 10–15 minutes. Furthermore, the equipment is transportable and the investigation can be performed at the patient's bedside or while anaesthetic preparations are underway.

The fitness of the patient for surgery requires detailed assessment of the various organ systems including cardiac, respiratory, renal, and blood and coagulation profile (see Ch. 2).

INDICATIONS FOR SURGERY

In an asymptomatic individual, the indications to perform elective repair of the thoracic aorta are based on an assessment of the risk of rupture or a complication versus operative risk. Unlike the natural history studies that are available for infrarenal abdominal aortic aneurysms (Szilagyi et al 1966), there are no comparable studies for thoracic aortic aneurysms. An analysis of aortic diameter of patients presenting with leakage and rupture reveals an increased risk for those aneurysms over 5 cm in diameter. Thus, in a good-risk patient with an asymptomatic thoracic aneurysm larger than 5 cm in diameter, elective repair is advisable provided the surgeon can perform this with an acceptably low morbidity and mortality. It is important to emphasize that the size considerations mentioned above apply to fusiform aneurysms. Saccular aneurysms are prone to rupture irrespective of size and present a more pressing indication for prophylactic surgery.

Surgery for an emergency presentation of thoracic aortic pathology carries a much higher morbidity and mortality risk. None the less, acceptable salvage rates can still be achieved provided the patient has no gross organ dysfunction or has not had a prolonged cardiac arrest prior to arrival at the hospital.

ANAESTHESIA FOR THORACIC AORTIC ANEURYSMS

Anaesthesia for thoracic aortic surgery presents additional problems over and above that of standard cardiac or vascular surgery. The metabolic insults suffered by the patient during extensive, prolonged surgery emphasize the importance of preoperative preparation. Major stress during the surgery and postoperative phase occurs on the cardiovascular system, respiratory system and renal systems.

Cardiovascular drugs should be selected in association with a cardiologist to minimize the risk of cardiovascular stress during anaesthesia and surgery. In particular, hypertension should be well controlled, prior to and during surgery, and a regimen designed to control hypertension and pain after surgery.

Lung function requires careful evaluation. Patients require either a median sternotomy or thoracotomy, depending on the nature of the operative procedure. In both cases, preoperative respiratory therapy by a physiotherapist and possibly antibiotic and bronchodilator therapy may be necessary. No elective surgery should be performed before the respiratory status is optimized.

Renal failure is a common cause of morbidity in thoracic aortic surgery. Postoperative renal failure requiring dialysis or filtration is associated with mortality of 45% or greater. If there has been a recent aortogram, elective surgery should be delayed until the serum creatinine has returned to the patient's normal level because of the risk of precipitating renal failure. Attention to hydration prior to surgery will help eliminate the prerenal causes of renal failure. Whilst it is not proven therapy, most teams use mannitol, low-dose dopamine and frusemide infusion during surgery in an attempt to reduce the risk of postoperative renal failure.

Special aspects of anaesthesia for aortic surgery

Patients presenting for aortic surgery can be divided into emergent or elective. Most emergency cases will present following haemorrhage or dissection. These patients exhibit varying degrees of shock and perhaps cardiac tamponade. Cardiac tamponade can be diagnosed preoperatively with a

transoesophageal echocardiogram. The echocardiogram features of tamponade are the presence of fluid in the pericardium and diastolic collapse of the right atrium. The Doppler findings in tamponade include a fall in left ventricular outflow tract velocity by at least 25% and a decrease in transmitral flow by at least 25% and increase in flow across the tricuspid valve by at least 25% during inspiration. If tamponade is present, induction of anaesthesia is particularly hazardous. Anaesthesia tends to remove vasoconstriction and blunt the onset of tachycardia, thus removing the compensatory mechanisms which occur during tamponade. Anaesthesia may result, therefore, in acute cardiovascular collapse and death. In such cases, aspiration of the pericardium is often unreliable. Intubation and groin cannulation under local anaesthesia together with simultaneous induction of anaesthesia and institution of partial cardiopulmonary bypass appears to be the preferred technique. In the period prior to institution of bypass, the anaesthetist must endeavour to prevent periods of hypertension because these may precipitate further bleeding and hypoxia.

Once anaesthesia is induced, both elective and emergency thoracic surgery present similar problems. All patients require standard care for cardiac surgery but, in addition, certain aspects need special consideration. These include airway control, monitoring, fluid replacement, clotting disorders and hypothermia.

Airway control
Airway control depends on the type of procedure. Single-lumen tubes are satisfactory for surgery to the ascending aorta and arch. Procedures on the descending thoracic aorta surgery require placement of a double-lumen tube. In descending thoracic aortic surgery, trauma to the left lung is

common and a double-lumen tube is required so that lung trauma is minimized. Should the aneurysm rupture into the left bronchus, a double-lumen tube protects the right bronchial tree from blockage with blood.

If possible, a left double-lumen tube is preferred. However, the presence of a haematoma in the area of the left bronchus may make this very difficult. In such cases, a right double-lumen tube may be used, provided the anaesthetist is able to ventilate the right upper lobe of the right lung.

Monitoring
Monitoring of haemodynamic parameters is essential. In addition to normal open-heart monitoring, blood pressure monitoring and blood gas sampling are necessary in these prolonged procedures. Surgery on the aortic arch requires use of arterial lines in both arms and, if possible, in the opposite foot to the femoral bypass. A dorsalis pedis line is mandatory in descending aortic surgery.

Fluid replacement
Fluid replacement is critical in all phases of management of patients having aortic surgery. Massive blood loss, occurring rapidly and suddenly, may be a feature of aortic surgery. Adequate vascular access for rapid transfusion is essential. In addition to one or two intravenous lines in the arm, multiple-lumen catheters[1] which are now available are useful. Such catheters can be sited in the internal jugular vein prior to induction of anaesthesia, at the same time as insertion of the Swan–Ganz catheter. In elective surgery, this line can be used for removal of autologous blood or platelet rich plasma (p. 19).

---

[1] Arrow-Howes™ Large-Bore Multi-Lumen Central Venous Catheterization Set, Arrow International, Inc., 3000 Bernville Road, Reading, PA 19605, USA.

During surgery, the use of a cell saver (p. 21) can limit the requirement for donor blood transfusion.

Hypothermia

Severe hypothermia with resultant bleeding and risk of ventricular fibrillation is an additional problem. Attention to warming intravenous fluids, raising the temperature of the operating room and airway heating with humidification are important. However, it is still not uncommon for patients to finish surgery with a temperature of 32°C. The recently available BAIR Hugger[TM][2] has proven useful in reversing hypothermia. The system consists of a warming unit which blows warmed air over the patient via a blanket. The chances of burning the patient are minimal as the heating mechanism is by convection using warm air. Attention to the areas outlined should improve survival in this most challenging area of anaesthesia and surgery.

[2] BAIR Hugger[TM], Augustine Medical, Inc., 10393 West 70th Street, Eden Prairie, MN 55344, USA.

SURGICAL APPROACHES

Median sternotomy

The median sternotomy is performed in the standard fashion with the exception that the superior extent of the skin incision is carried well into the suprasternal notch to allow maximal exposure superiorly. After opening the chest retractor and suspending the pericardium with stay sutures, aortic mobilization is commenced. The amount of external mobilization around the aorta is kept to a minimum to reduce the risks of rupturing the aneurysm or dislodging atheromatous debris. The repair can be achieved most easily by working within the aortic lumen rather than attempting to perform a complete mobilization. None the less, a few manoeuvres have been found to be useful. Firstly, the aorta is separated from the pulmonary artery by incising the aortopulmonary groove (Fig. 5.1a). Secondly, the pericardium is reflected off the right side of the ascending aorta and off the anterior surface of the aorta and pulmonary artery. Downward retraction on the ascending aorta together with upward retraction of the left innominate vein will expose the base of the innominate artery and left common carotid (Fig. 5.1b). No attempt is made to dissect the arch vessels completely or encircle them with tape. The next important manoeuvre is the clearing of the left lateral and inferior surface of the aortic arch (Fig. 5.1b). It is important to stay close to the adventitia of the aorta to avoid injury to the left phrenic nerve as it crosses the arch anterior to the left pulmonary artery under cover of the pericardium. As this dissection proceeds along the lateral surface of the aortic arch, a few small unnamed arteries are found arising directly off the arch which require control with diathermy.

Left thoracotomy

Patient positioning is critical. This begins by ensuring that a 'bean bag' has been placed underneath the warming blanket. The patient is placed in the right lateral position, making sure that the patient's back is at the edge of the table. The chest should be at 90° to the table. If distal perfusion via the femoral artery is to be used, it is important to allow the pelvis to rotate up to about 45° from the horizontal. The upper arm is supported on the overhead arm rest and secured to it with a crêpe bandage. The right leg is flexed at the hip and knee, while the left leg is kept straight and a pillow is inserted between the two legs. The patient may be secured with tapes. However, it is important to ensure that the tape does not interfere with access to the femoral artery. Suction on the bean bag further stabilizes the patient's position. All pressure points must be adequately padded, particularly the dependent axilla, ulnar and common peroneal nerves.

The middle portion of the skin incision is placed approximately two fingers' breadth below the tip of the scapula and from there extends forward in a direction which depends on the desired intercostal access required. For instance, if a fourth intercostal space incision is desired, the anterior part of this incision can be curved forward into the inframammary crease. If, on the other hand, there is a possibility of extending the incision into a thoracoabdominal one, it can be curved downwards in a lazy 'S' to follow the sixth or seventh ribs to the costal margin. The posterior portion of the incision curves upwards to lie halfway between the medial edge of the scapula and the spinous processes. Once again, its proximal extent depends on the desired intercostal space, but it will generally require extension to the level of the spine of the scapula. After the incision has reached to the dermis, further dissection is carried out with diathermy to minimize subsequent chest wall bleeding. The latissimus dorsi is divided in the anterolateral portion of the incision as is the lower edge of the trapezius posteriorly. The next layer consists of the serratus anterior, which is incised as low as possible to retain its innervation. More posteriorly, and in the same layer, are found the rhomboid muscles. After incision of these layers, it is possible to slide a heavy retractor under the scapula and to locate the desired intercostal space by counting downwards from the first rib.

Generally, the approach to the distal arch and proximal descending aorta requires entry into the fourth intercostal space, while for the mid and distal descending aorta the fifth or sixth space is chosen. The 'bucket handle' incision may also be used to gain access to the whole descending aorta by entering two different intercostal spaces.

The incision into the intercostal space is made along the upper edge of the rib with diathermy, ensuring complete haemostasis. In addition, in order to enhance exposure, a small segment of the posterior end of the rib below the intercostal incision is resected. A chest retractor is inserted and slowly opened to avoid causing a rib fracture. The left lung is allowed to collapse at this stage and any adhesions between the lung and chest wall or mediastinum are divided.

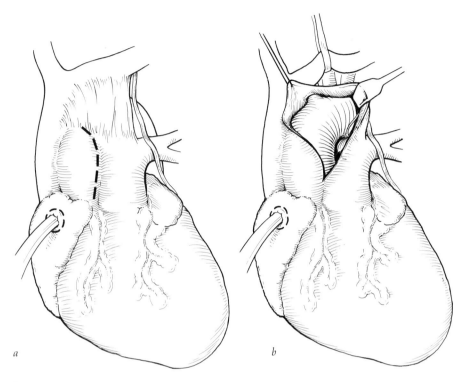

a   *b*

Fig. 5.1
Exposure of the ascending thoracic aorta and aortic arch through a median sternotomy.

Aortic mobilization is commenced by making a longitudinal incision in the mediastinal pleura overlying the anterlateral surface of the descending aorta and extending proximally over the arch and then continuing upwards over the left subclavian artery (Fig. 5.2a). The left superior intercostal vein will be found crossing the arch underlying this incision and will require ligation and division. It is vital to deepen this incision to the correct perivascular plane close to the aorta before attempting any further mobilization. The anteromedial surface of the aorta is cleared by sweeping the pleura and the vagus nerve medially. The insertion of the ligamentum arteriosum into the underside of the arch is then located and divided (Fig. 5.2b). This allows the mediastinal tissue containing the vagus and recurrent laryngeal nerve to fall away from the underside of the arch towards the midline. It is now possible to carry this dissection around the posterior aspect of the arch. Turning now to the pleural incision over the left subclavian artery, the mediastinal pleura is swept medially, exposing the superior surface of the arch in the angle between the left subclavian and left common carotid arteries. The lateral lip of the mediastinal pleura over the subclavian artery is retracted laterally and the left subclavian artery can be completely encircled. It is essential in this part of the dissection to stay within the perivascular plane because a more superficial dissection encircling the subclavian artery risks injury to the thoracic duct and subsequent chylothorax.

Distal mobilization of the descending thoracic aorta is performed at the desired level by incising the pleura longitudinally over the aorta. The pleura is retracted laterally, while an assistant gently retracts the aorta medially. With this manoeuvre, the intercostal vessels can be seen readily

and encircled if necessary. If there is difficulty in finding the intercostal arteries, the necks of the adjacent ribs are palpated to determine the intercostal space which is followed medially to the intercostal artery. The aorta is mobilized medially by retracting the medial leaf of the pleural incision and the aorta encircled using a curved vascular clamp rather than a finger, which can avulse the intercostal arteries from the aorta.

HAEMOSTASIS AND BLOOD CONSERVATION

Both intraoperative and postoperative haemorrhage are a major source of morbidity and mortality after thoracic aortic surgery. Problems with haemostasis are contributed to by a number of factors, including systemic heparinization, a prolonged cardiopulmonary bypass time, hypothermia, extensive dissection and multiple suture lines. The recent appreciation of the role of platelet dysfunction resulting from activation of the fibrinolytic system has been instrumental in understanding haemostatic defects following cardiopulmonary bypass. Contact between blood and a foreign surface activates both the coagulation cascade and the fibrinolytic mechanism, which results in the production of plasmin. Plasmin damages the glycoprotein receptors on the platelets, resulting in impairment of platelet aggregation and degranulation. Heparin inhibits the coagulation cascade but does not affect activation of the fibrinolytic mechanism.

A major development in diagnosis of haemostatic defects has been the Thromboelastograph[R] (TEG[TM3]) (Hartert 1948). The TEG gives a

quantitative measure of viscoelastic clot strength. The clot strength is transduced to a paper write-out or computer screen and several classical patterns are easily recognized (Fig 5.3). In particular, it is easy to diagnose primary fibrinolysis and to follow its treatment with ε-aminocaproic acid or similar antifibrinolytic drugs. This TEG can be used within an operating room to detect the most common causes of haemostatic failure, namely platelet dysfunction and fibrinolysis. Abnormalities on the TEG are evident before the standard tests of haemostatic function such as platelet count, activated partial thromboplastin time and prothrombin ratio show any abnormalities. The use of this procedure reduces the need for laboratory back-up.

Management of bleeding disorders begins with prophylaxis. It is appropriate to wait until the effects of aspirin, anti-flammatory agents or warfarin wear off before undertaking elective surgery. It is vital to have access to an adequate supply of blood and blood products: 10—20 units of blood, fresh frozen plasma and platelets are cross-matched routinely. The platelet units are pooled in one bag to allow rapid transfusion. An important adjunct is the use of preoperative plasmapheresis to obtain platelet-rich plasma. If this technique is not available, then, prior to heparinization and cardiopulmonary bypass, withdrawal of 0.5—1 litre of autologous blood is a useful alternative.

In view of the central role that fibrinolysis plays in platelet dysfunction, an antifibrinolytic agent such as aprotinin or ε-aminocaproic acid is administered. It is important to deliver this agent prior to the onset of the cascade effect otherwise large quantities of the antifibrinolytic agent are required to neutralize the activated plasmin. The development of collagen-impregnated woven grafts (p. 126) has been useful. The traditional densely woven

---

[3] Haemoscope Corporation, 5836 Lincoln Avenue, Morton Grove, IL 60053, USA. © 1991 Haemoscope Corporation TEG and Thromboelastograph.

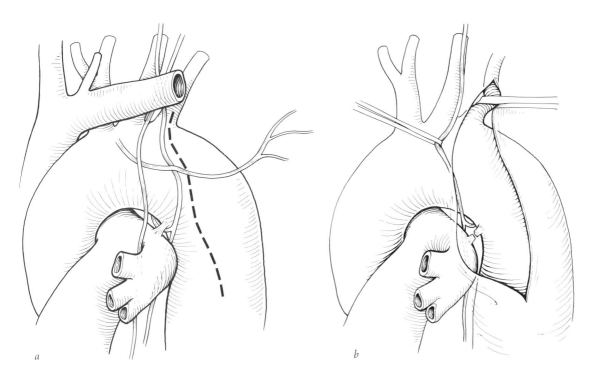

a

b

Fig. 5.2
Exposure of the distal
aortic arch through
the chest.

non-porous grafts are difficult to handle,
while the collagen-impregnated grafts
have minimal porosity and are very
compliant. Topical haemostatic agents
such as Surgicel ©,[4] topical thrombin
and fibrin glue (Guilmet et al 1979) can
minimize the bleeding from large raw
surfaces.

Surgical haemostasis is paramount
because continued bleeding from a
surgical defect can cause rapid
consumption of coagulation factors and
a secondary coagulopathy which is
difficult to reverse even with large
quantities of blood and blood products.
The intraoperative use of cell saver
(p. 21) helps conserve red blood cells
lost prior to heparinization or after
reversal with protamine. It also allows
salvage of the blood remaining in the
cardiopulmonary bypass pump. Red
blood cell salvage continues in the
postoperative phase with the use of
retransfusion of mediastinal drainage.

[4] Surgicel ©, Johnson & Johnson Ltd, Trade Mark
code 53812: Ethicon, PO Box 408, Bankhead Ave.,
Edinburgh EH11 4HE, UK.

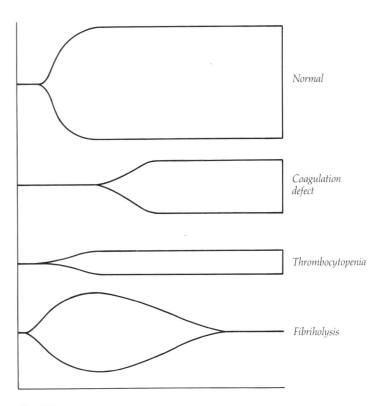

Normal

*Coagulation
defect*

Thrombocytopenia

Fibriholysis

Fig. 5.3
Thromboelastograph® patterns of coagulation and platelet abnormalities.

Coagulopathy is treated specifically according to the results of coagulation tests and thromboelastography. Thrombocytopenia or platelet dysfunction is treated with platelet transfusion. Desmopressin has not been found useful in situations of platelet dysfunction, with the exception of patients with chronic renal failure and in those with von Willenbrand's disease. Coagulation factor deficiencies are treated with fresh frozen plasma and cryoprecipitate.

BYPASS TECHNIQUES

The need for and type of bypass is determined by the management of blood flow proximal and distal to and that arising from branches of the excluded segment of the aorta. This is best discussed by dividing the aorta into three segments: aortic root and ascending, arch and thoracoabdominal.

As the ascending aorta carries the whole cardiac output, replacement of this segment requires full cardiopulmonary bypass. For similar reasons, replacement of the aortic arch also requires full bypass, but with the added burden of providing cerebral flow. While this may be achieved by arch vessel cannulation, a more practical solution is the use of deep hypothermia and circulatory arrest.

Multiple options are available for the thoracoabdominal aorta. These include simple clamping and pharmacological manipulation of the circulation, partial bypass around the excluded segment, and deep hypothermia and circulatory arrest (see p. 46).

Cardiopulmonary bypass via median sternotomy

This approach is used for repair of aneurysms or diseases of the aorta extending from the aortic valve through the aortic sinuses, ascending aorta and proximal aortic arch. For pathology confined to the aortic valve sinuses and proximal ascending aorta, the cannula for the arterial return can be placed in the distal ascending aorta or proximal arch as illustrated in Figure 5.4. If the disease involves most of the ascending aorta or arch then femoral arterial return is required (Fig. 5.5). Venous cannulation is by a standard two-stage right atrium catheter (Fig. 5.4), or with a longer venous cannula threaded from the right femoral vein into the right atrium (see Fig 5.6, p. 47). The latter approach is preferred in complex cases as it reduces the amount of tubing in the operative field. It is also essential when there has been acute leakage or rupture, where cardiopulmonary bypass needs to be instituted prior to opening the chest, and when retrograde cerebral and vital organ perfusion is to be used. Femoral cannulation can be life saving in a reoperation where it is suspected that the aorta is adherent to the inner table of the sternum. A retrograde coronary sinus catheter is routinely placed for the administration of cardioplegia solution.

Deep hypothermia and circulatory arrest

Each tissue has a critical time during which it can survive without circulation, by drawing on its own energy reserves. This limited time before the onset of irreversible tissue damage is referred to as the 'safe period' of circulatory arrest. The brain is the most sensitive tissue because of its limited capacity for anaerobic metabolism. As most energy consumption in tissue is secondary to enzymatic processes and since the activity of enzymes is temperature dependent, one may logically use hypothermia to prolong the 'safe period'. The metabolic rate of human tissues drops by a factor of 2.5 for each 10°C drop in temperature. Hence the safe period of circulatory arrest can be graphed against temperature, as illustrated in Table 5.1.

Table 5.1 The basal metabolic rate (BMR) and oxygen consumption and period of safe circulatory arrest (CA) as a function of body temperature (T)

Temperature (°C)	BMR/VO$_2$ (%)	CA (min)
37	100	4–5
29	50	8–10
22	28	16–20
16	12	30–45
10	6	60–80

Injury to the central nervous system is related to the depth of hypothermia and the duration of circulatory arrest. In clinical series, circulatory arrest periods of up to 45 minutes at temperatures at or below 20°C have not been associated with any neurological deficits. Between 45 and 60 minutes, transient diffuse impairment in the form of drowsiness, inability to concentrate and a flat affect which reverses spontaneously in a few days is common. Beyond 60 minutes, there is increasing risk of permanent diffuse neurological injury with coma and death.

Other factors that affect the likelihood of cerebral injury are the rates of cooling and rewarming. The temperature gradient between the water bath in the heat exchanger and the patient's temperature should not exceed 10°C because gas may come out of solution during rewarming and cause microembolism. Metabolic factors include the adjustment of pH and blood glucose during hypothermia. As tissues are cooled, the point of pH neutrality increases. Attempts to maintain the pH at 7.40 at low temperatures results in tissue acidosis, impairment of cerebral autoregulation and predisposes to central nervous system injury. Hyperglycaemia promotes metabolism via the glycolytic pathway with generation of lactate and intracellular acidosis and so should be avoided. There is no convincing evidence that the use of drugs such as steroids and barbituates has any major impact on the development of cerebral complications.

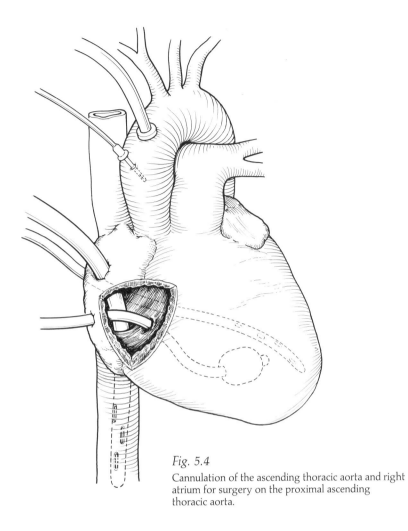

Fig. 5.4
Cannulation of the ascending thoracic aorta and right atrium for surgery on the proximal ascending thoracic aorta.

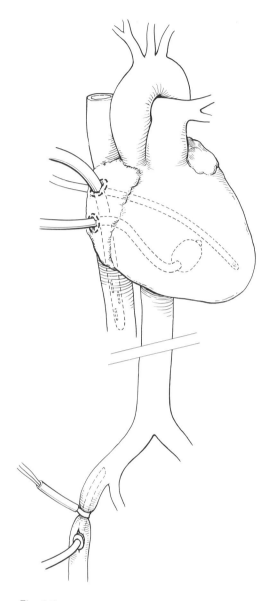

Fig. 5.5
Cannulation of right common femoral artery and right atrium for surgery involving the distal ascending thoracic aorta and arch.

Controversy surrounds the optimal temperature for hypothermia and circulatory arrest. During cooling, there can be as much as a 10°C difference or more between various sites used for measuring the temperature such as the nasopharynx, oesophagus, tympanic membrane, rectum and bladder. It is probable that the nasopharyngeal and tympanic membrane temperatures more closely approximate brain temperature than the other sites. The EEG has been used to relate the bypass temperature to a reduction in cerebral activity. Crawford et al (1987) have recommended that cooling should continue until electrical activity on the EEG disappears irrespective of the temperature.

Techniques of deep hypothermia and circulatory arrest

Deep hypothermia and circulatory arrest can be used when the approach is through a median sternotomy, a left thoracotomy or thoracoabdominal incision. The cannulation technique when the approach is from a median sternotomy is shown in Figure 5.6. Arterial return is through a femoral artery cannula and venous outflow is from a long venous cannula introduced via the right femoral vein and positioned with its tip in the right atrium. Occasionally, the femoral vein catheter will not pass the site where the right common iliac artery crosses the left common iliac vein and distal inferior vena cava. A useful manoeuvre to help negotiate this obstruction is to introduce a size 8-French nasogastric tube which has been threaded through the lumen of the venous cannula or ahead of the venous cannula as shown in the inset of Figure 5.6. The tip of the nasogastric tube will negotiate the obstruction and help guide the venous cannula into position. This arrangement of venous cannulation greatly improves visibility and access in the chest and can be readily adapted to the technique of retrograde IVC and SVC perfusion (see Fig. 5.7). A coronary sinus catheter is inserted through the right atrium for delivery of retrograde cardioplegia. Bypass is instituted and cooling commenced.

In the cases of severe aortic regurgitation, there may be a problem with left ventricular (LV) distension despite the presence of an LV vent, or there may be difficulty in maintaining adequate systemic flow and pressure. In these circumstances, it may be necessary to cross-clamp the ascending aorta. The clamp is applied preferably to a segment of aorta which is going to be replaced. Cardioplegia is given for the duration of the aortic cross-clamping and circulatory arrest.

Once aortic exposure and dissection are complete and the degree of cooling required has been reached (we cool to a temperature of 16–18°C depending on the anticipated duration of circulatory arrest), the patient is placed head down and the pump is turned off. The patient's blood volume drains into the reservoir. It is important that during the period of circulatory arrest a steep, head-down (Trendelenburg) position is maintained, so that a pool of blood remains in the cerebral vessels. The arch vessels should not be aspirated dry because of the risk of intraining air into the cerebral vessels, resulting in embolization when the circulation is reinstituted.

Once the repair of the aorta has been completed, the pump is turned on very slowly so that the blood ascending from the descending thoracic aorta can displace any air in the arch or great vessels. Atheromatous debris that had been dislodged from the aortic wall during the surgical procedure will float on the top of the rising air blood level and can then be removed. At the completion of this process, the graft is clamped and full pump flow is reinstituted.

Retrograde superior vena cava perfusion and retrograde inferior vena cava perfusion

This technique, which is still at its early stages of development, attempts to provide continuous cerebral and other vital organ perfusion during the period of circulatory arrest by delivering retrograde perfusion via the superior and inferior venae cavae (Matalanis & Buxton 1993). The main aim is to reduce the degree of hypothermia required to permit safe antegrade circulatory arrest. This in turn will reduce the time required for cooling and rewarming and will possibly reduce the associated coagulopathy. In addition, the continuous retrograde perfusion may provide protection against air and

particulate emboli. If this technique provides adequate cerebral and vital organ perfusion, it may allow extension of the antegrade circulatory arrest period beyond the 1-hour limit and also permit the conduct of circulatory arrest at warmer temperatures.

The arterial and femoral cannulation is as described for deep hypothermia and circulatory arrest. In addition to the usual retrograde coronary sinus catheter, a second retrograde catheter is placed via the right atrium into the superior vena cava (Fig. 5.7). The superior vena caval junction with the right atrium is dissected and encircled with tape. The bypass circuit is also modified by placing a shunt between the main arterial and venous pump lines (Fig. 5.7). Cardiopulmonary bypass is instituted and the patient cooled to 20°C. Antegrade perfusion is discontinued and the tape surrounding the superior vena caval junction is snugged around the retrograde cerebral catheter, and retrograde cerebral perfusion is commenced (Fig. 5.8). Generally, pump flows at 150–600 ml/min are maintained with careful attention to the perfusion pressure, which is maintained below 30 mmHg. The inferior vena cava cannula is withdrawn to below the diaphragm and a clamp is applied to the junction of the inferior vena cava and the right atrium (Fig. 5.8). Retrograde inferior vena cava perfusion is then commenced by diverting arterial blood to the main venous line as illustrated.

At the conclusion of the distal end of the repair, the retrograde cerebral perfusion is continued in order to displace any air in the graft or head vessels. The graft is then clamped and the retrograde perfusion discontinued. The tape around the superior vena cava and the clamp at the junction of the inferior vena cava with the right atrium are removed and the inferior vena cava cannula advanced back into the right

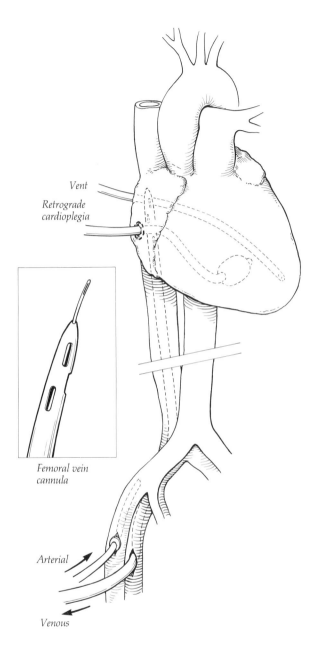

Fig. 5.6
Cannulation of the right common femoral artery and vein for extensive proximal aneurysms, emergencies and deep hypothermic circulatory arrest.

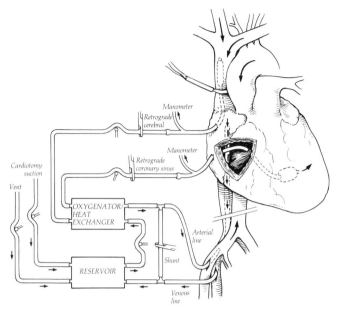

Fig. 5.7
Cannulation and circuit diagram for deep hypothermic circulatory arrest combined with retrograde superior vena cava and inferior vena cava perfusion.

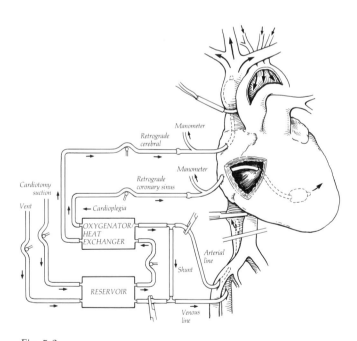

Fig. 5.8
Circuit diagram and technique of retrograde coronary sinus, superior vena cava and inferior vena cava perfusion (Matalanis & Buxton 1993).

atrium. The bypass circuit is then restored to its original form and antegrade perfusion recommenced.

Partial left heart bypass from the left chest

The goal of distal aortic perfusion is to unload the proximal circulation and provide distal perfusion for the spinal cord, kidneys and other viscera.

The methods of distal perfusion can be classified into passive and active shunts. The latter can also be subclassified into those that use a reservoir and oxygenator and those that do not.

Passive shunts take the form of temporary or permanent bypass grafts or, more commonly, tube shunts such as the Gott shunt. The advantages are simplicity, ready availability and the avoidance of systemic heparinization because of the heparin-bonded tube. This is particularly important in the context of multiple trauma and central nervous system injury. On the other hand, the disadvantage is that there is no active control over the flow, this being entirely dependent on a pressure gradient between the upper and lower half of the body and the resistance of the tube. Even the largest tube imposes significant resistance to flow. The only safe means of using these shunts is in concert with a flow meter and a femoral artery pressure line.

Active shunts as a group have the advantage of using cannulae which are large enough not to provide significant resistance to flow. In addition, flow can be controlled precisely. Finally, the incorporation of a heat-exchange circuit allows the ability to cool or warm the patient. The centrifugal pump with a heparin-bonded circuit is an active shunt without reservoir or oxygenator. This circuit requires minimal or no heparinization. However, it has no reservoir and therefore it is not possible to return scavenged blood directly to the circuit. It also lacks an oxygenator, hence its inflow has to be from an oxygenated source such as the left atrium or proximal aorta. Active shunts

with an oxygenator and/or reservoir, on the other hand, require full heparinization and so may increase the risk of bleeding and are contraindicated in multiple trauma where there is a possibility of abdominal or neurological injury. Alternatively, they provide the benefit of oxygenation.

Cannulation techniques

Systemic veins such as the femoral vein can be used for outflow. The advantage is easy accessibility and low morbidity, but a pump oxygenator is required. Another outflow site is the left atrium via its appendage. This contains oxygenated blood and hence there is no need for an oxygenator although a pump is required. However, the left atrium is friable and can tear easily. In addition, cannulation may be associated with atrial fibrillation and the risk of air embolism. The left ventricular apex as an outflow site has the advantage of blood being oxygenated and at systemic pressure. However, there are major disadvantages such as the risk of haemorrhage and development of a false aneurysm, the risk of ventricular fibrillation and air embolism. Finally, if used in combination with a passive shunt, there is a 30–40% reduction in flow when compared to the ascending aorta as an outflow site. Furthermore, there is a 15% reverse flow ('aortic regurgitation') during diastole. The proximal aorta, either the ascending or arch, can be used as an outflow site providing oxygenated blood at normal pressure. However, access to the proximal aorta may be very difficult in the presence of a large descending aortic aneurysm. Also, the aorta is often diseased and cannulation may cause dissection or thromboembolism.

Inflow for many of the distal perfusion techniques is usually via the femoral artery. However, if this is extensively diseased, then the iliac artery or the abdominal aorta may be used.

The left atrial to femoral arterial left heart bypass is the distal perfusion technique of choice, as illustrated in Figure 5.9a. An angled venous cannula is placed through the left atrial appendage into the left atrium (Figure 5.9b, c). This drains to a centrifugal (Biomedicus®)[5] pump which directs flow back into the lower half of the body through a left femoral artery cannula. A heparin-bonded circuit can reduce the systemic heparin requirements. Flow is directed around the segment of aorta excluded by the cross-clamps. Flow rates are adjusted to achieve unloading of the proximal aorta, and at the same time supplying a distal aortic perfusion pressure of at least 60 mmHg.

It is important to remember that with any of the distal perfusion techniques to date, there is no conclusive evidence that they consistently lower the incidence of paraplegia or renal impairment. They are all associated with the possibility of cannulation site morbidity. There are circumstances in which their use is difficult, such as the presence of aorto-iliac occlusive disease or the presence of an extensive thoracoabdominal aneurysm requiring replacement to the aortic bifurcation. In addition, in an emergency, with acute leakage or perforation, there may be no time to institute these measures. Finally, it is important to realize that all of these methods provide no direct assistance to the proximal circulation, which is entirely dependent on continuous cardiopulmonary function.

---

[5] Biomedicus® Medtronics, 9600 West 76 Street, Eden Prairie, Minneapolis, MN, USA.

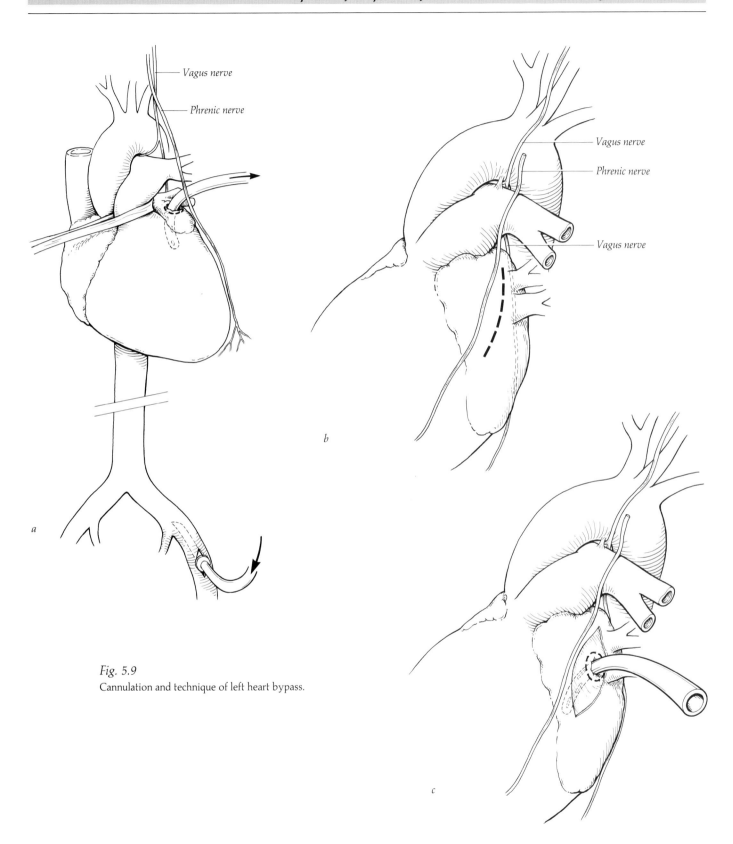

Fig. 5.9
Cannulation and technique of left heart bypass.

Deep hypothermic circulatory arrest from the left chest

Deep hypothermia and circulatory arrest from the left chest may be used when it is undesirable to place a proximal clamp on the ascending aorta. Indications include very large aneurysms, reoperation where access for clamping proximal to the aneurysm is unavailable, or where the aorta is heavily calcified or atheromatous.

Cannulation is shown in Figure 5.10. The arterial return is to a left femoral arterial catheter. Venous drainage is through a long venous cannula placed in the left common femoral vein which is positioned with the tip high in the right atrium. If the venous drainage is inadequate, or if it is impossible to introduce the venous catheter beyond the iliac bifurcation, a second cannula should be placed in the pulmonary artery.

Difficulties and special problems
Deep hypothermic circulatory arrest from the left chest can present special problems. Some patients require cannulation of the right femoral vein either as a supplement or as the sole venous drainage because of potential difficulty in obtaining satisfactory venous drainage from the left side.

The prevention of distension of the heart during ventricular fibrillation is more difficult and is best managed by ensuring adequate venous drainage and, if necessary, inserting a vent in the main pulmonary artery through the pericardial sac.

Cerebral protection is also more difficult from the left side. It is not possible to use retrograde cerebral perfusion in this position and the potential for cerebral embolism is very real.

The sequence of clamp removal and flushing of the major arteries is very

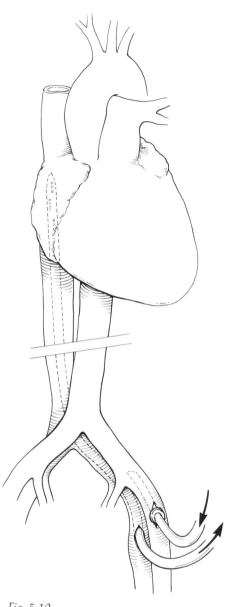

Fig. 5.10
Cannulation of the left femoral artery and vein for deep hypothermic circulatory arrest from the left chest.

important. Whenever releasing a clamp, it is vital that the distal pressure should be lower than the proximal, in case embolic material is dislodged from a distal atheromatous aorta into the cerebral circulation.

SPINAL CORD ISCHAEMIA

The risk of spinal ischaemia with paraparesis or paraplegia after operations on the descending and thoracoabdominal aorta is related to a number of factors.

Aortic pathology
In cases of coarctation with a well-developed collateral system, the risk of paraplegia is under 0.5%. In operations for aortic dissection, where all the intercostal vessels are patent and without a collateral circulation, the risk is high and is twice that for surgery on an atherosclerotic aneurysm.

Site of the aorta which has been replaced
Resection of the proximal and middle thirds of the descending aorta is associated with paraplegia risk of less than 3%, while replacement of the distal third of the descending aorta has a risk of about 8%.

The length of aorta replaced
Replacement of the entire aorta from the left subclavian to the bifurcation is associated with a 30% risk of spinal cord ischaemia, while replacement of the whole abdominal aorta is only associated with about 2% risk.

Occurrence of perioperative hypotension
This may be related to an emergency presentation with rupture, or intraoperative hypotension related to loss of control during mobilization or declamping. Postoperative hypotension is associated with bleeding or occurrence of low cardiac output.

A number of ancillary procedures have been devised in an attempt to lower the risk of paraplegia, but there is no agreement that any one of these results in a lower incidence of paraplegia.

The pathophysiology of spinal cord ischaemia relates to the peculiarity of the anatomy of its blood supply. The anterior spinal artery supplies the anterior half to two-thirds of the spinal cord. This artery, which begins in the brain stem, becomes very narrow and discontinuous in the lower third of the thoracic segment. Continued perfusion of the spinal cord below this point is dependent on radicular branches from intercostal and lumbar arteries. In the human, there may be two to five radicular branches, the major one being called the artery of Adamkiewicz, and this is the major source of blood flow to the distal spinal cord. In 75% of cases this artery arises from a left intercostal artery between the segments of T9 and T12.

Although most cases of paraplegia are due to ischaemia, additional injury to the spinal cord may be caused by reperfusion injury, the occurrence of a spinal haematoma and conduction of electrical current from diathermy close to the dural sheath of the intercostal nerves.

Spinal cord ischaemia may be prevented in several ways. The ischaemic injury to the cord can be reduced by limiting cross-clamp time to 30 minutes, avoiding general hypotension, increasing the distal aortic pressure by distal perfusion, avoiding the use of nitroprusside, reimplantation of important intercostal arteries, cerebrospinal fluid drainage (Crawford et al 1990), and anterior spinal artery dilatation with intrathecal papaverine. Reperfusion injury can be reduced by the use of calcium channel blockers, free radical blockers and steroids. Another approach is to try to slow the metabolic rate of the spinal cord and thus prolong the safe ischaemic time by the use of either topical hypothermia in the chest or systemic deep hypothermia and circulatory arrest. Finally, some have attempted to provide an alternative

source of oxygen for the spinal cord by perfusing the intercostal arteries or by direct intrathecal perfusion of fluosol.

One of the problems with reimplantation of the intercostal arteries is how to select the appropriate arteries. The likely sites for the artery of Adamkiewicz are intercostal arteries between the level of T9 and T12, especially on the left side. Also, intercostals that have a wide orifice and poor back-bleeding should be implanted. Preoperative localization with selective angiography is associated with a number of false positives and negatives and also may cause paraplegia. Intraoperative localization has been attempted by the use of somatosensory-evoked potentials and motor-evoked potentials and more recently by the intraoperative perfusion of hydrogen into isolated aortic segments (Svensson et al 1990). Unfortunately all of these techniques are unreliable. Furthermore, there are certain disadvantages of intercostal artery reimplantation such as prolongation of cross-clamp time, the risk of intraoperative or postoperative thrombosis of the reattached artery and the possibility of early haemorrhage from the intercostal artery anastomosis or the development of late aneurysms at the site of reimplantation.

In those patients who develop paraplegia postoperatively, approximately half will have total and severe paralysis with loss of bladder and bowel control. These patients tend to make a poor recovery and have an associated 30% perioperative mortality. The other half have partial leg weakness with a retention of bladder and bowel control and they generally make a good recovery. Although in about 80% of cases the paraplegia is present at the time of awakening from anaesthesia, another 20% occur in the 3 weeks after surgery postoperatively. The paraplegia tends to have a spinal level of about T8

(costal margin) with preservation of light touch due to posterior column preservation.

Despite all the measures, paraplegia remains a major problem following repair of the descending thoracic aorta. The correct monitoring of proximal and distal arterial pressures, the avoidance of hypovolaemia, the use of bypass techniques and preservation of the major intercostal arteries will help minimize the risk of paraplegia, which increases with the distal extent of the resection. Evoked sensory potentials and motor potentials, CSF decompression and H_2 monitoring are currently being evaluated and may have a role in the future in identifying which intercostal arteries should be preserved.

REFERENCES

Barbetseas J, Crawford S, Safi H J, Coselli J S, Quinones M A, Zoghbi W A 1992 Doppler echocardiographic evaluation of pseudoaneurysms complicating composite grafts of the ascending aorta. Circulation 85: 212–222

Chan K L 1991 Usefulness of transesophageal echocardiography in the diagnosis of conditions mimicking aortic dissection. American Heart Journal 122: 495–504

Crawford E S, Coselli J S, Safi H J 1987 Partial cardiopulmonary bypass, hypothermic circulatory arrest, and posterolateral exposure for thoracic aneurysm operation. Journal of Thoracic and Cardiovascular Surgery 94: 824–827

Crawford E S, Svensson L G, Hess K R et al 1990 A prospective randomized study of cerebrospinal fluid drainage to prevent paraplegia after high-risk surgery on the thoracoabdominal aorta. Journal of Vascular Surgery 13: 36–46

Erbel R, Engberding R, Daniel W, Roelandt J, Visser C, Rennollet H 1989 Echocardiography in diagnosis of aortic dissection. Lancet i: 457–460

Guilmet D, Bachet J, Goudot B et al 1979 Use of biological glue in acute aortic dissections: a new surgical technique. Preliminary clinical results with a new surgical technique. Journal of Thoracic and Cardiovascular Surgery 77: 516–521

Hartert H 1948 Blutgerinnung studein mit der thrombelastographie, einen neuen untersuchingsverfahren. Klinische Wochenschrift 26: 577–583

Matalanis G, Buxton B 1993 Retrograde vital organ perfusion during aortic arch repair. Annals of Thoracic Surgery 56: 981–984

Nienaber C A, Spielmann R P, von Kodolitsch Y et al 1992 Diagnosis of thoracic aortic dissection: magnetic resonance imaging versus transesophageal echocardiography. Circulation 85: 434–447

Svensson L G, Patel V, Coselli J S, Crawford E S 1990 Preliminary report of localisation of spinal cord blood supply by hydrogen during aortic operations. Annals of Thoracic Surgery 49: 528–536

Szilagyi De, Smith R F, DeRusso F J, Elliott J P, Sherrin F W 1966 Contribution of abdominal aortic aneurysmectomy to prolongation of life. Annals of Surgery 164: 678–699

Chapter 6

Aneurysms of the thoracic aorta

Brian Buxton   George Matalanis

THORACIC AORTIC ANEURYSMS

The frequency of thoracic aortic aneurysms is increasing along with the age of the population. The surgical treatment of aneurysms and dissections of the thoracic aorta, once a surgical curiosity, is now becoming commonplace and there is no area of the aorta which is not readily accessible for surgical correction. This change in attitude to the management of diseases of the thoracic aorta is due partly to improvement in surgical technique, but perhaps more importantly to the development of innovative strategies for preservation of the brain, spinal cord and other vital organs during the obligatory interruption of the normal circulation to these structures (Borst et al 1964, Borst 1981, Matalanis & Buxton 1993).

Investigations

The management of patients presenting urgently or as an emergency with rapid enlargement, leakage, rupture or dissection of a thoracic aneurysm requires minimal delay and the avoidance of unnecessary investigations and transport. The investigations are directed to confirming the diagnosis and determining whether or not the aneurysm or dissection is best approached through a median sternotomy or a lateral thoracotomy. Transoesophageal echocardiography is almost ideal as it requires minimal preparation and it can be used without transferring the patient. Angiography is used to confirm the presence and site of a traumatic rupture.

The assessment of patients presenting electively is directed at determining the site and length of the aorta involved and the diameter of the aorta at different levels. The size of the aorta can be measured accurately with echocardiography, computed axial tomography (CT) and magnetic resonance imaging. Angiography is best for defining the anatomy of the aortic branches.

Follow-up of any surgical procedure is essential because aneurysmal dilatation in one area may herald dilatation in another. The diameter of adjacent segments of the thoracic aorta can be measured by transoesophageal echo or CT at repeated intervals to follow the progress of the non-grafted segments.

Surgical techniques

The surgical techniques available for correction of aneurysms of the thoracic aorta will be described in conjunction with the preferred method of vascular access or cannulation and a description of the most appropriate circuit for the particular procedure.

ASCENDING THORACIC AORTIC ANEURYSMS

Tube graft repair of the ascending thoracic aorta using an aortic cross-clamp

This procedure is confined to those ascending thoracic aneurysms which terminate proximal to the innominate artery leaving a cuff of normal aorta which allows a clamp to be placed so that there is enough aorta for the distal suture line. If it is not possible to clamp the distal ascending thoracic aorta, deep hypothermic circulatory arrest can be used, thus avoiding the use of the cross-clamp (see p. 46). Tube graft repair may be used for aneurysms involving the aortic root, but an aortic root repair should be used when aneurysms are associated with connective tissue disorders because any residual aortic root may undergo further dilatation.

The procedure is performed through a standard median sternotomy incision with reflection of the pericardium at the upper end to gain access to the terminal extrapericardial section of the ascending thoracic aorta for cannulation (Fig. 6.1).

Arterial cannulation is performed either in the distal ascending thoracic aorta (Fig. 5.4) or common femoral artery (Fig. 6.1). Venous drainage is usually possible through the right atrium unless the aneurysm is of very large proportions, when venous drainage is more easily obtained through the right common femoral vein with a long venous cannula extending into the right atrium (Fig. 5.6). A vent is placed in the left ventricle through the right superior pulmonary vein and left atrium for decompression of the heart during this procedure.

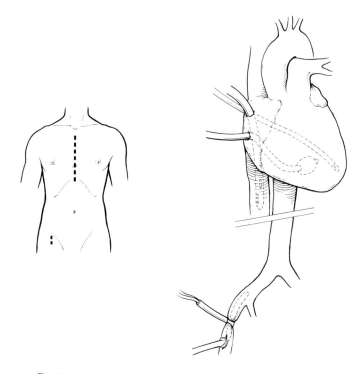

Fig. 6.1
Tube graft repair of ascending thoracic aorta.

Once on cardiopulmonary bypass, the aorta is cross-clamped. The aorta is then opened longitudinally on its anterior surface over the extent of the aneurysm (Fig. 6.2a, b). The inner surface of the aorta is inspected carefully. The point of transection is chosen at the distal end of the aneurysm where the aorta resumes a normal diameter. The transection may be partial or complete if access is difficult. Care should be taken when the aorta is completely divided to avoid damage to the right and main pulmonary artery. The proximal extent of the aneurysm is defined and, if the aortic root is not involved, the aorta is divided either completely or partially above the level of the coronary arteries.

A graft is chosen to match the diameter of the aorta. The graft is then transected with scissors or electrocautery, slightly obliquely if necessary so that the circumference of the graft will match that of the proximal aorta.

The graft is sutured proximally to the aortic root with a running, long-length, monofilament suture commencing in the aorta at the point opposite the surgeon, above the commissure between the left and right coronary cusps. The suture is then continued around the posterior wall, terminating in the region of the non-coronary cusp (Fig. 6.2c). The other limb of the suture is brought around the anterior wall of the aorta above the right coronary artery, which must be carefully avoided. Special care must be taken to produce good apposition during suturing along the posterior wall, particularly if it has not been transected, because this is relatively inaccessible once the operation has been completed. The sutures should be positioned accurately and appropriate tension maintained throughout the suture line.

Prior to performing the distal anastomosis, the graft is put under tension and divided, leaving a little extra length so that the graft can be elevated later to check haemostasis on the posterior aspect of the upper and lower suture lines at the end of the procedure. Again, the anastomosis commences on the left side of the aorta and continues to the right along the posterior wall and subsequently around the right wall of the aorta for a variable distance (Fig. 6.2d). The second suture is then brought around the left wall of the aorta and across the anterior wall towards the right. Before completing the distal suture line, the left ventricular vent is turned off, the heart filled with blood and air evacuated by massage of the ventricle. The suture is tied and a needle inserted through the dacron graft at its highest point. The aortic clamp is released gradually to remove the remaining air from the aorta through the vent needle, which is subsequently connected to suction. This needle is left on suction until a normal cardiac output has been established and all air has been evacuated. Once a normal arterial pressure has been re-established, both suture lines are checked for bleeding. When this is completed, the redundant tissue in the aneurysm sac is resected and the remaining sac is loosely wrapped around the dacron graft to isolate it from the sternum (Fig. 6.2e). This is not intended to be haemostatic. The patient is removed from cardiopulmonary bypass and the cannulation sites oversewn.

Tube graft repair of the ascending thoracic aorta and aortic root (Wheat technique)

This operation (Wheat et al 1964) is similar to that described above except for the proximal suture line. It is indicated where there is aneurysmal dilatation of the ascending thoracic aorta involving the aortic root, particularly in the region of the non-coronary sinus. This operation is contraindicated in patients with connective tissue disorders such as Marfan's disease, where the remaining aortic wall may undergo further dilatation requiring a secondary procedure. The aortic valve may need replacement if there is significant aortic regurgitation. However, an aortic root replacement may be preferable if there is significant annular dilatation.

Surgical technique
The surgical approach, cannulation and bypass circuit are the same as in the previous section.

The aorta is opened longitudinally, extending proximally into the region of the aortic root. The aorta is transected proximally, leaving a small rim of tissue adjacent to the aortic annulus except in the region of the coronary artery orifices, where the incision leaves the region of the annulus and passes superiorly over the coronary artery orifice and then returns to the region of the annulus in an inverted 'U' fashion. If there is moderate or severe aortic regurgitation, the aortic valve is replaced separately.

The graft is trimmed to match the contour of the aortic wall, with additional material being removed from the graft in the region of the left and right coronary artery orifices. The suture line usually commences towards the left side, staying away from the left coronary artery orifice, and then continues around the posterior wall to the right side of the aorta (Fig. 6.2f). The second needle is then used along the anterior wall of the aorta, looping up in the region of the right coronary artery orifice and the anastomosis is completed at the right margin of the aorta.

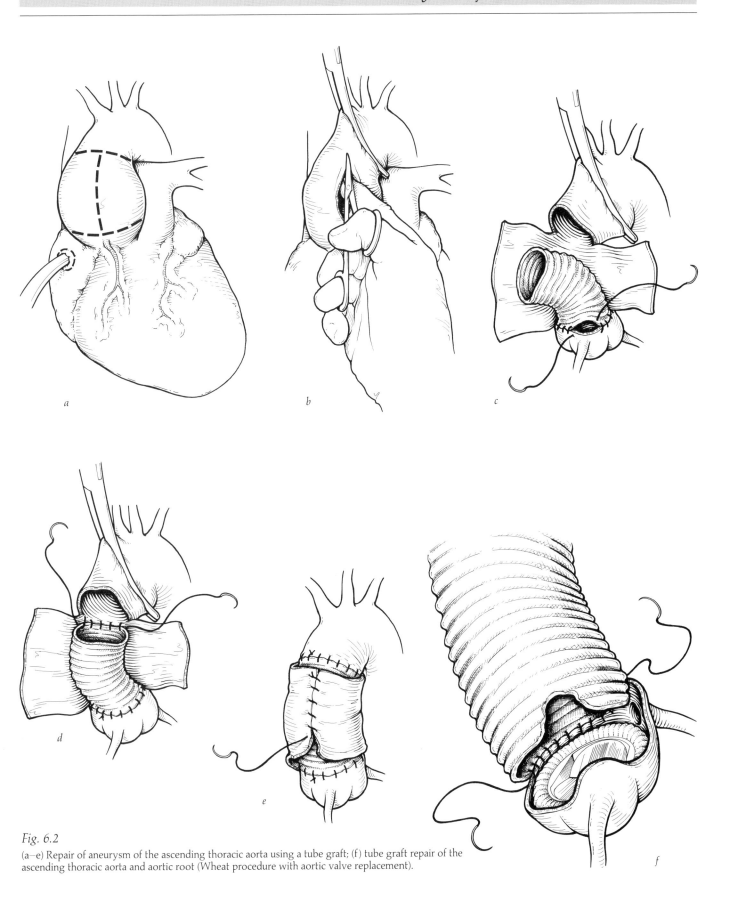

Fig. 6.2

(a—e) Repair of aneurysm of the ascending thoracic aorta using a tube graft; (f) tube graft repair of the ascending thoracic aorta and aortic root (Wheat procedure with aortic valve replacement).

Repair of the aortic root and ascending thoracic aortic aneurysm using a valve conduit

We believe that this operation should be restricted to well-defined pathological conditions involving the aortic root, although the general trend is to use a composite valve conduit for any pathology of the aortic root. A common indication is annuloaortic ectasia in which there is a localized connective defect involving the aortic root with dilatation of all three sinuses and upward displacement of the coronary artery orifices (Zubiate & Kay 1976). The operation should be used also in any patient with an aneurysm of the ascending thoracic aorta who has a connective tissue disorder such as Marfan's disease or Ehlers–Danlos syndrome, where a less extensive operation leaving aortic root tissue behind often results in further dilatation, requiring a secondary procedure. The routine use of this operation for aneurysms of the proximal ascending thoracic aorta or aortic root will result in the unnecessary loss of a normal aortic valve or a valve which could be repaired. With the exceptions mentioned, every effort should be directed to performing a conservative procedure preserving the aortic valve.

The approach, cannulation and bypass techniques are similar to those for tube graft replacement of the ascending thoracic aorta. Several commercial types of valve conduits are available. The ordinary graft is porus and therefore will require preclotting to prevent excessive blood loss in the heparinized patient. This can be achieved by preclotting the graft with albumin sprayed onto the graft. A small swab is placed over the valve to protect it from any albumin spilling into the region of the valve and valve hinge. As the albumin is placed on the graft, the graft material is stretched to impregnate the pores. The valve conduit is autoclaved to coagulate the protein and render the graft non-porous. If this step is omitted, it is possible to neutralize the heparinized blood with protamine and apply this blood to the graft in a similar way to the albumin without the use of the autoclave.

Bentall procedure (Bentall & De Bono 1968)

The aorta is opened longitudinally along the anterior surface of the aorta and the exposure is increased by a short transverse incision at either end to display the aorta, aortic root and its contents (Fig. 6.3a). In patients with dilatation of the aortic root, the exposure of the aortic valve is usually very good. Stay sutures are placed in each commissure and the valve leaflets excised, leaving a small rim of valve tissue. The valve annulus is measured with a valve sizer. The diameter of the distal ascending thoracic aorta is also measured. Obtaining the correct size of the valve conduit is important. In general, the size of the valve annulus takes priority over the size of the distal aorta. It is, however, possible to place a slightly smaller aortic valve, if the conduit appears excessively large for the distal aorta. The valve conduit is then sutured into the aortic annulus with interrupted 2/0 multifilament sutures with small teflon pledgets placed either above or below the aortic annulus (Fig. 6.3a). These sutures are passed through the prosthetic valve ring prior to lowering the valve into position. Subannular placement of the sutures and pledgets will bring the coronary arteries slightly closer to the aortic wall than with the supra-annular pledget technique (Fig. 7.4e, f).

The left coronary artery orifice is identified and the relationship to the adjacent dacron graft is noted. If the aortic wall is pliable, the coronary artery orifice is sutured in situ using the graft inclusion technique (Kouchoukos 1991). If tension exists, the risk of suture line dehiscence is unacceptable and mobilization of the coronary artery orifice with a small button of aortic wall is preferred. A small circular opening about 5–6 mm in diameter is made in the dacron graft using a hand-held electrocautery with the graft displaced inferiorly (Fig. 6.3b). The left coronary artery orifice is sutured to the opening in the dacron with a running 4/0 monofilament suture commencing at the left end and working towards the right on the inferior wall and again on the anterior wall (Fig. 6.3c). It is important to obtain a double thickness of the aorta with each of these sutures to prevent suture-line dehiscence and secondary aneurysm formation.

The graft is then tilted towards the head to expose the right coronary artery orifice and an opening is made in the graft for the anastomosis (Fig. 6.3d). Again, if the aorta is pliable and reaches the graft easily, it can be sutured in situ. The anastomosis is performed with a running monofilament suture starting from the left end, obtaining thick bites of the aortic wall immediately adjacent to the coronary artery itself (Fig. 6.3e).

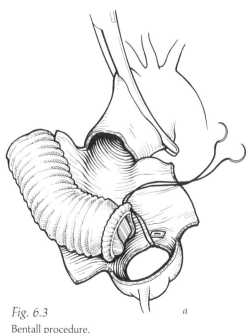

Fig. 6.3
Bentall procedure.

a

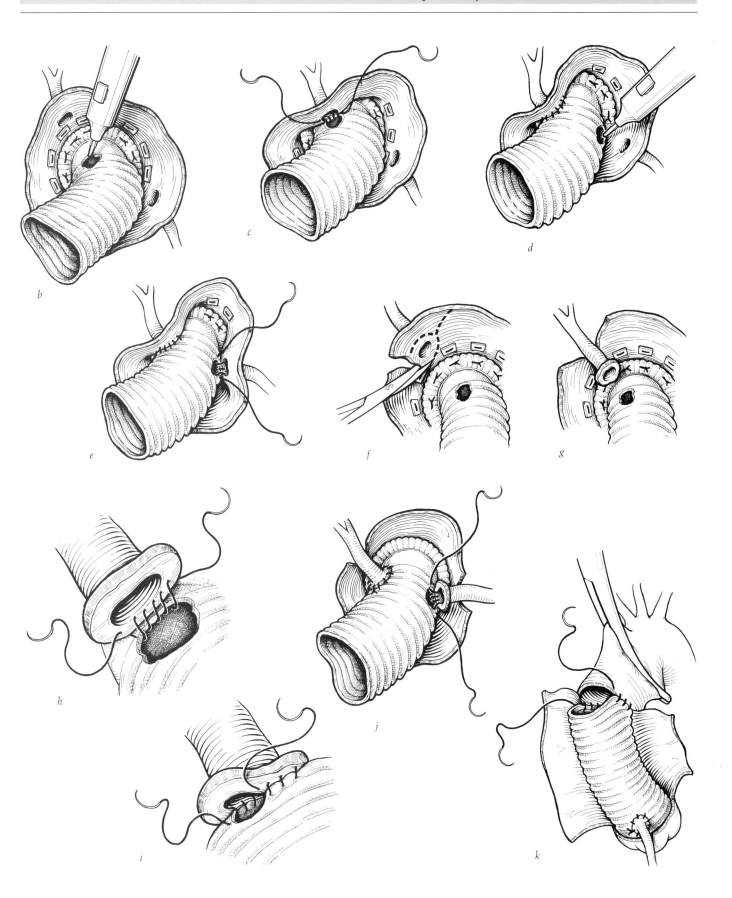

An accessory coronary artery orifice such as that of the conus branch should be included with the main right coronary artery in this anastomosis.

In recent years, the technique of using the coronary artery with a button of aortic wall technique has been more popular than the in situ anastomoses because of ease of access, the ability to secure haemostasis and the prevention of late false aneurysms. The left coronary artery is mobilized with sharp dissection, with a cuff of aortic wall extending about 4–5 mm from the coronary artery orifice (Fig. 6.3f). The incision is deepened and the coronary artery mobilized for approximately 0.5–1 cm (Fig. 6.3g). During this mobilization, it is important to be aware that occasionally the left main coronary artery is very short and the circumflex branch can be damaged. If divided, direct repair with interrupted fine sutures is usually satisfactory. Similarly, when mobilizing the right coronary artery the conus branch can be injured but this may be oversewn without myocardial damage. The anastomoses between the mobilized coronary arteries with the surrounding aortic wall are performed in the same way as with the in situ technique. To ensure a good haemostatic suture line it is better to take a second bite of the aortic wall with each of the sutures (Fig. 6.3h–j). It is easier to repair a leak in the posterior left coronary to dacron graft anastomosis than when the in situ technique is employed. If any doubt exists about the haemostasis, cardioplegia solution can be introduced through the dacron graft to check the coronary artery suture lines. With the increased use of retrograde cardioplegic solution, this step is often omitted.

The distal anastomosis is then performed between the dacron graft and the distal ascending thoracic aorta with a monofilament suture (Fig. 6.3k). Haemorrhage between the aneurysm sac and the graft can result in excessive tension on the coronary artery suture lines, resulting in a false aneurysm. A loose wrap of the aneurysm sac which is not intended to be haemostatic is therefore recommended in most situations.

Special difficulties
Coronary arteries are usually elevated in patients with a connective tissue disorder of the aortic root and therefore the anastomosis between the dacron graft and the coronary arteries is relatively straightforward. In some patients, however, if the coronary artery orifices are in the normal or low position, the suture lines are more difficult and require greater mobilization of the coronary arteries. If it is not possible to perform a direct suture between the coronary artery and the dacron graft, the Cabrol technique (Fig. 7.7a–d) (Cabrol et al 1981) or a bypass graft may be necessary to restore normal flow to the left or right coronary artery.

If the graft inclusion technique has been used and there is tension in the space between the graft and the aneurysm sac, secondary decompression is possible by anastomosing the right atrial appendage to the aneurysm sac (Cabrol et al 1981).

ASCENDING THORACIC AORTA AND ARCH ANEURYSMS

Aneurysms of the aortic arch are uncommonly found in isolation, usually occurring in association with aneurysms of the ascending thoracic aorta or the upper descending thoracic aorta. Rarely, degenerative aneurysms of the saccular type may be localized to the aortic arch. The arch can be the site of traumatic rupture or dissection (see Fig. 7.8a–c).

The indications for surgery are similar to those of the ascending or descending thoracic aorta and are based primarily on the aneurysm size or the onset of complications.

Preservation of cerebral function and other vital organ function is the main challenge to the surgeon correcting disease involving the aortic arch. The use of deep hypothermic circulatory arrest developed in paediatric cardiac surgery and adapted by Borst et al (1964), for aortic aneurysm surgery, greatly simplifies the approach to surgery involving the aortic arch which hitherto involved complicated bypass circuits or temporary bypass grafts to the cerebral vessels (Liversay et al 1982, Crawford et al 1989). Deep hypothermic circulatory arrest has certain limitations which have been discussed earlier in Chapter 5.

Repair of aneurysms of the ascending thoracic aorta and proximal aortic arch using deep hypothermic circulatory arrest
The ascending thoracic aorta and proximal aortic arch are exposed through a standard median sternotomy with additional dissection of the proximal arch. The innominate vein is mobilized from the aortic arch and elevated with slings.

Arterial cannulation is by the right common femoral artery, with venous drainage through the right common femoral vein using a single long venous cannula with the tip placed in the atrium. Occasionally, an additional superior vena cava cannula is required if the venous drainage is inadequate. A coronary sinus catheter is used for retrograde cardioplegia, while a left ventricular vent is inserted through the right superior pulmonary vein passing through the left atrium. Our practice now includes additional cerebral protection with retrograde cerebral perfusion (Ch. 5, p. 46). A further coronary sinus catheter is placed in the superior vena cava via the right atrium for retrograde cardioplegia. A sling is passed around the vena cava proximal to the catheter balloon (see Fig. 5.7).

After appropriate cooling and arresting of the circulation, the aortic arch is opened longitudinally, extending from the aortic root to the proximal aortic arch. The aortic exposure is improved by a transverse incision at the upper and lower limits of the aortic incision (Fig. 6.4a). Retrograde cerebral perfusion is commenced by using a separate arterial pump, the flow being regulated to about 150–600 ml/min and limited by a pressure of 30 mmHg. During this perfusion, blood emerges from the arch vessels and is removed from the distal aortic arch by a separate cardiotomy sucker. Another refinement is to perfuse the abdominal organs and spinal cord retrogradely, via the inferior vena cava (see Ch. 5).

Surgical repair
A graft of the appropriate size is anastomosed distally to the aorta immediately beyond the aneurysm using a continuous suture (Fig. 6.4b). Once this anastomosis is completed, the retrograde cerebral and organ perfusion is discontinued and the femoral-to-femoral bypass recommenced very slowly. The aortic graft is left open so that any atheroma, other particulate debris or air is evacuated from the graft (Fig. 6.4c). The graft is then cross-clamped to direct the flow to the brain and the remainder of the body (Fig. 6.4D) except the heart, which is still protected by the retrograde cardioplegia. The proximal end of the dacron graft is divided again, leaving sufficient length for subsequent inspection of the posterior suture line. The anastomosis is commenced on the left side and continued posteriorly and is then completed anteriorly (Fig. 6.4d). Before closure of the lower aortic anastomosis, the vent is stopped and the heart and the lungs are inflated so that blood is directed from the ventricle through the aortic opening, which is

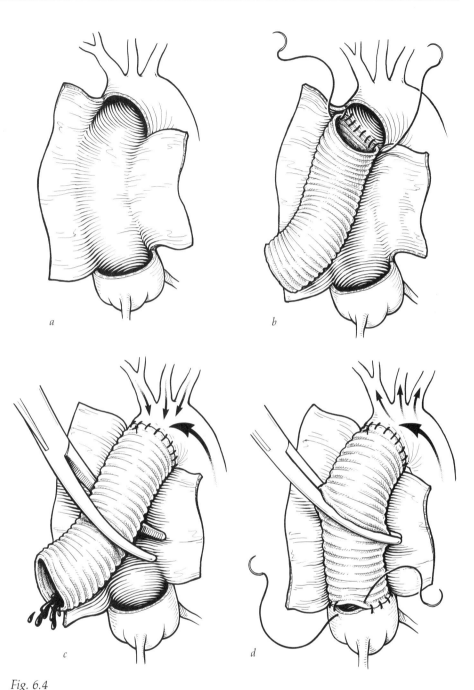

Fig. 6.4
Repair of aneurysms of the ascending thoracic aorta and proximal arch using deep hypothermic circulatory arrest.

subsequently closed. A vent is placed in the proximal aortic graft and the aortic cross-clamp is subsequently released slowly. The posterior suture line is examined carefully for bleeding and the aneurysm sac wrapped loosely over the dacron graft.

Repair of an aneurysm involving the ascending thoracic aorta and aortic arch

Aneurysms of the ascending thoracic aorta with extensive involvement of the entire aortic arch are approached from a median sternotomy using deep hypothermic circulatory arrest (see p. 46) with the same bypass technique as described above (Figs 5.7 and 5.8).

Exposure of the aortic arch is obtained by mobilizing the innominate vein and continuing the dissection around the anterior and left side of the aortic arch in a plane close to the aorta, displacing the phrenic and the vagus nerves laterally. Mobilization of the innominate, left common carotid and subclavian arteries is kept to a minimum because it is not necessary to isolate, control and clamp these arteries using deep hypothermia. The aorta is partly transected at the distal end and everted (Fig. 6.5a, b). A dacron graft is chosen to match the size of the distal aorta and sutured using continuous monofilament suture commencing inferiorly and proceeding along the posterior wall to a point distal to the left subclavian artery orifice (Fig. 6.5c). The anastomosis of the graft to the anterior wall of the upper end of the descending thoracic aorta is completed. The graft is put on tension and an oval window of the graft removed from the superior surface adjacent to the aortic arch vessels (Fig. 6.5d). A continuous suture is commenced distally and the posterior layer completed before commencing the anterior layer which completes the single anastomosis incorporating the innominate, common carotid and left subclavian arteries (Fig. 6.5e). The femoral arterial perfusion is recommenced slowly so that all air is displaced from the major arteries and embolic material is directed through the opened end of the dacron graft (Fig. 6.5f). Once removal of the debris is complete, the retrograde cerebral

perfusion is discontinued. The graft is clamped and antegrade flow is restored to the brain and abdominal viscera (Fig. 6.5g). The proximal reconstruction is completed as above.

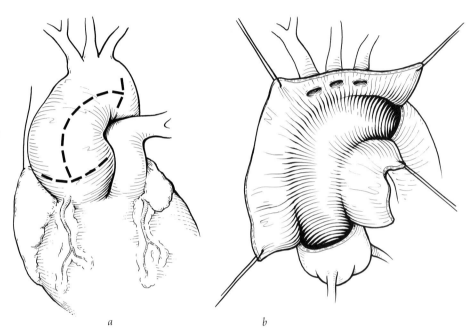

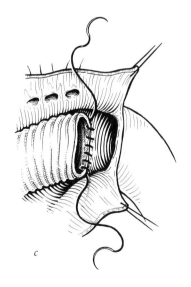

Fig. 6.5
Repair of aneurysm of the ascending thoracic aorta and aortic arch.

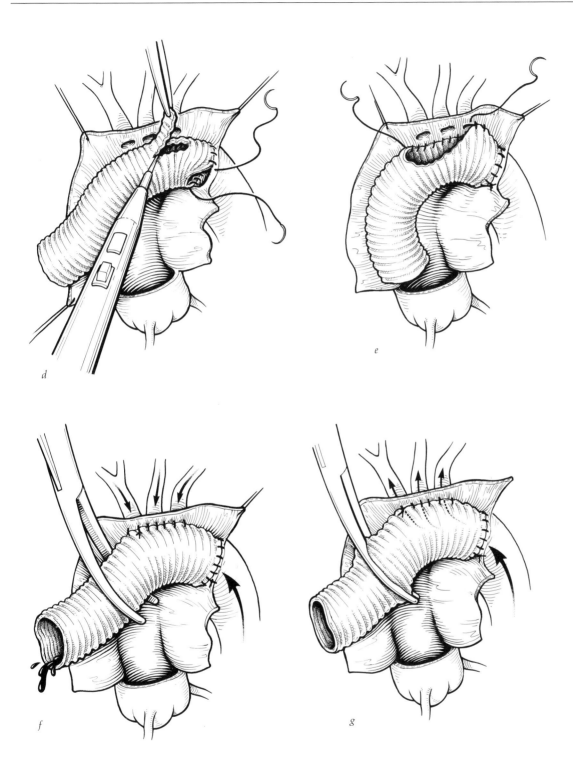

Repair of inferior wall of the aortic arch

This technique is used when there is aneurysmal dilatation of the inferior wall of the aortic arch with minimal aneurysmal dilatation involving the arch vessels and superior surface of the aortic arch.

The operation is similar to that described previously, except there is a single oblique distal anastomosis incorporating the upper descending thoracic aorta and arch vessels. The dacron graft is stretched and cut in an 'S'-shaped fashion (Fig. 6.5h) to correspond to the oblique suture line in the ascending aortic arch.

The posterior suture line is commenced at the most distal point on the inferior wall of the upper descending thoracic aorta and continued posteriorly and to the right, passing obliquely across the aortic arch (Fig. 6.5i). The anterior suture line encloses the descending thoracic aorta and three arch vessels to complete anastomosis (Fig. 6.5j). The proximal end of the graft is sutured to the aortic root (Fig. 6.5k).

Aneurysms of the aortic root, ascending thoracic aorta and aortic arch

Complex aneurysms involving this entire segment are handled in a way similar to aneurysms of the arch described previously up to the point where the bypass is recommenced and the aortic graft has been clamped after removal of any embolic material. Attention is returned to the aortic root where the appropriate surgical procedure is performed, for example as described in Figures 6.2 or 6.3 during rewarming of the patient. If there is annular dilatation and aortic root disease, a valve conduit is implanted into the aortic root with interrupted multifilament sutures and teflon pledgets. The coronary arteries together with a small rim of aortic wall are mobilized and sutured with a continuous monofilament suture. The valve conduit and the distal dacron graft are orientated and the length measured and then trimmed. The two dacron grafts are joined using monofilament suture (Fig. 6.5l). Before completion of this anastomosis, air is removed from the heart and an aspiration needle is left in the proximal aorta to complete the evacuation of air before release of the aortic clamp.

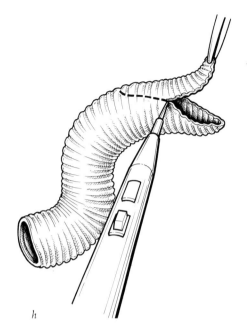

h

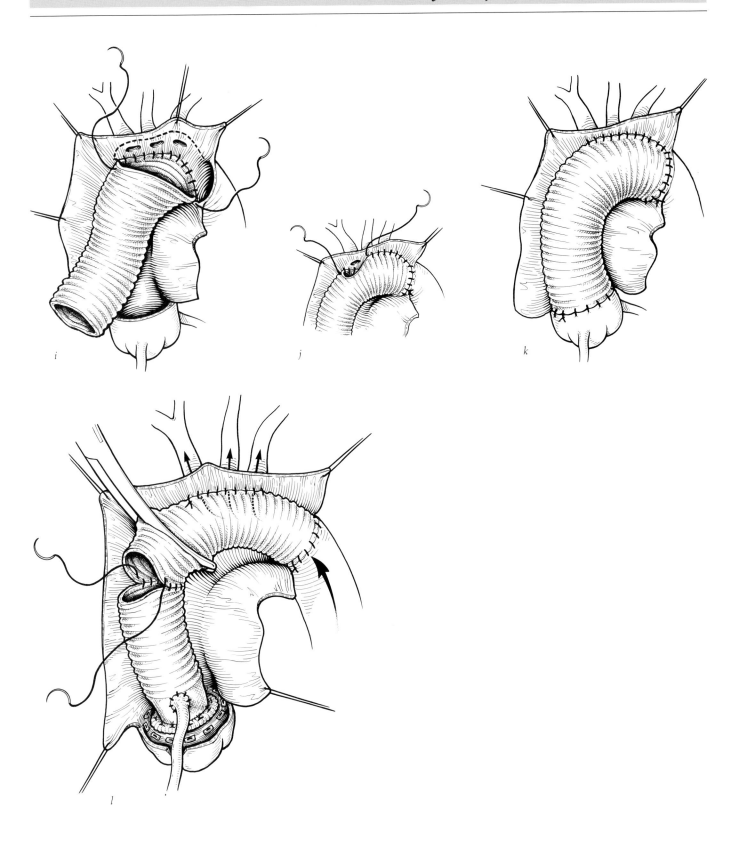

Mega aorta—the elephant trunk procedure: stage I

Ascending thoracic aneurysms are frequently delineated from aneurysms of the descending thoracic aorta by a relatively normal-sized aortic arch. Aneurysmal dilatation involving the ascending thoracic, aortic arch and the descending thoracic aorta and onwards, thus involving the whole aorta, occurs sometimes, and is called the 'mega aorta'. Mega aorta also includes extensive chronic dissections of the aorta continuing through the arch into the descending thoracic aorta.

The elephant trunk procedure is an operation which, as a first stage, encompasses repair of the ascending thoracic aorta and arch. This first stage of the procedure greatly facilitates the upper end of the repair of the descending thoracic aorta which is performed as the second stage (Fig. 6.10, p. 74).

The operation proceeds in a way similar to the previous forms of aortic arch replacement using deep hypothermia and circulatory arrest.

The aortic arch is opened on its anterolateral surface, extending distally to the level of the subclavian artery (see Fig. 6.5b). A graft is then chosen to match the diameter of the aorta immediately distal to the left subclavian artery. The graft is intussuscepted, leaving a 4–5 cm length of dacron which will remain in the upper descending thoracic aorta (Fig. 6.6a). The distal anastomosis is performed to the double fold of the graft which has been placed in the distal aorta (Fig. 6.6b). On completion, the inner or intussuscepted layer of the dacron graft is withdrawn back into the aortic arch by forceps and the traction suture (Fig. 6.6c). The arch vessels are then anastomosed to the side of the dacron graft either individually or, preferably, as a single anastomosis (Fig. 6.6d). On completion of this anastomosis, the cardiopulmonary bypass is recommenced very slowly to displace air and particulate matter from the aortic graft and major arteries. If the graft in the upper descending thoracic aorta acts like a valve, preventing retrograde flow of the blood into the arch, a separate 8 mm dacron graft side arm is sutured to the main dacron graft to act as the arterial inflow site (Fig. 6.6e). After all air has been evacuated from the arch graft and retrograde flushing completed, the main graft is clamped and flow directed up the arch vessels into the distal descending thoracic aorta (Fig. 6.6f). If the aneurysm extends to involve the aortic root a separate graft is anastomosed to the aortic root (Fig. 6.6f, g). After removal of air is complete and haemostasis achieved, the small graft is divided and the stump oversewn. The sac is loosely approximated over the graft (Fig. 6.6h).

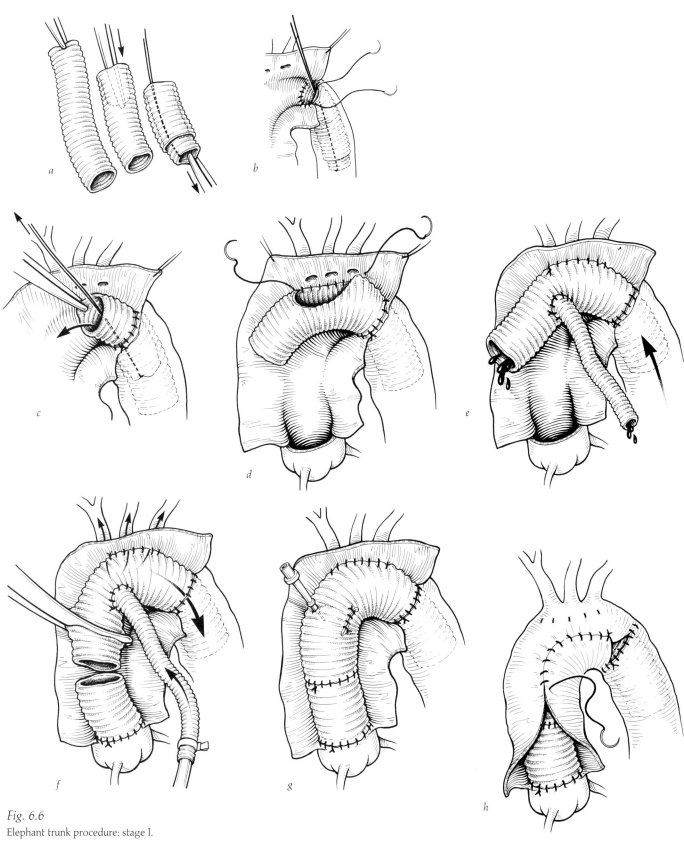

Fig. 6.6
Elephant trunk procedure: stage I.

DISTAL AORTIC ARCH ANEURYSMS

Distal aortic arch aneurysms involve the terminal part of the aortic arch and do not extend proximal to the left subclavian artery, so that they can be approached through the left chest. Two groups are identified: a more favourable group that can be managed by clamping the aortic arch between the left common carotid and left subclavian artery, and the other where access is more difficult and requires deep hypothermic circulatory arrest.

Distal aortic arch repair using aortic cross-clamp

Aneurysms involving the upper descending thoracic aorta with minimal extension into the arch can be treated by cross-clamping the aortic arch between the left subclavian and left common carotid with or without distal bypass. Post-traumatic aneurysms and some saccular aneurysms can be managed in this way. This approach is contraindicated in aneurysms where the access is difficult, the aortic tissue is friable or in those with numerous adhesions.

Surgical technique
The left chest is opened through a lateral thoracotomy using the fourth intercostal space. The patient is placed on left heart bypass by cannulation of the left atrial appendage for venous outflow and the left common femoral artery for arterial return (Fig. 5.9). The patient is maintained at normothermia. The vagus nerve is dissected from the lateral wall of the aorta and the ligamentum arteriosum divided, avoiding the recurrent laryngeal nerve (Fig. 5.2). The aortic arch is mobilized between the left subclavian and left common carotid artery and a sling placed around the aorta. The distal end of the aneurysm is identified and the pleura opened to display the aorta, which is encircled with tape.

Once the left heart bypass has been established (see p. 48), the aortic arch is cross-clamped between the common carotid and left subclavian artery and the distal descending thoracic aorta clamped below the aneurysm. The aneurysm sac is opened longitudinally and partially transected above and below the aneurysm (Fig. 6.7a). A graft is sutured end to end to the distal aortic arch using a running monofilament suture (Fig. 6.7b). A side hole is cut in the superior aspect of the main graft and the subclavian artery anastomosed either directly or with a short interposition graft to the side of the main graft using 4/0 monofilament sutures (Fig. 6.7b). The graft is stretched and divided at an appropriate place for the distal anastomosis. This is then performed with a running suture commencing medially and passing along the posterior wall of the anastomosis. The anastomosis is completed by suturing along the anterior wall (Fig. 6.7c). Before completion of the anterior layer of the anastomosis, the distal clamp is released to remove air or any embolic material from the descending thoracic aorta. The left subclavian clamp is also released to remove any embolic material from that vessel. Finally, the aortic arch clamp is released and the proximal aorta flushed gently. The proximal clamp can then be reapplied to the dacron graft distal to the subclavian artery and a vent needle placed in the graft to remove any residual air. The left heart bypass is discontinued and the proximal clamp released slowly. The suture lines are checked for bleeding and the aneurysm sac is loosely wrapped around the dacron graft.

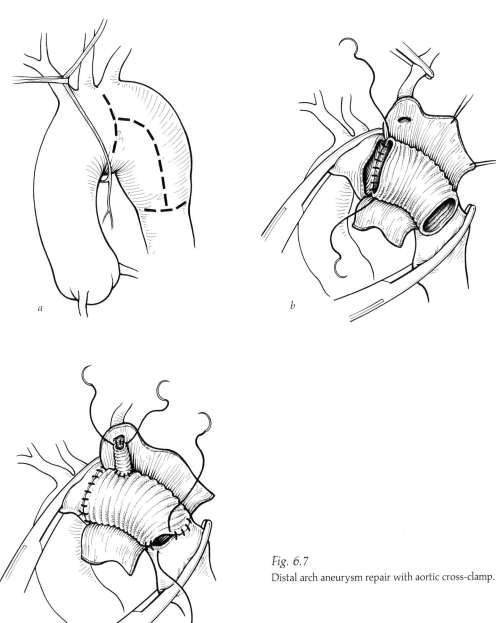

a

b

c

Fig. 6.7
Distal arch aneurysm repair with aortic cross-clamp.

Distal aortic arch repair using deep hypothermic circulatory arrest

More complex aneurysms of the distal aortic arch and upper descending thoracic aorta are best treated with deep hypothermic circulatory arrest without using clamps. The incision and surgical approach are the same as in the previous operation. Cannulation is through the left common femoral artery and vein. The patient is placed on full cardiopulmonary bypass and the temperature lowered slowly. The patient is placed in a 30° head-down position. When the required temperature is reached, normally 16–20°C, the bypass is discontinued and the venous drain is left open to produce exsanguination. The distal aortic arch and upper descending thoracic aorta is opened longitudinally and partially transected above and below the aneurysm. A graft is then anastomosed end to end to the aortic arch using a continuous monofilament suture (Fig. 6.8a). The left subclavian artery is anastomosed to the upper surface of the graft (Fig. 6.8b, c).

Alternatively, if the left subclavian artery cannot be brought directly down to the dacron graft a short interposition graft is required (Fig. 6.7c). The distal anastomosis is then performed between the main dacron graft and the descending thoracic aorta using a running monofilament suture. Prior to completion of the distal anastomosis, the cardiopulmonary bypass is recommenced very slowly to fill the aortic arch and cerebral vessels. After air and atheromatous debris have been removed, the suture line is closed and the cardiopulmonary bypass recommenced (Fig. 6.8d).

An alternative technique when the period of circulatory arrest is expected to exceed 60 minutes is to recommence the cardiopulmonary bypass after completion of the upper end using the 8 mm side arm, which is to be used for the subclavian reconstruction. This allows the distal anastomosis to be performed under cardiopulmonary bypass, thus minimizing the time of complete circulatory arrest (Fig. 6.8e). After the arterial line is joined to the 8 mm dacron graft, the cardiopulmonary bypass is commenced very slowly so that the air is displaced from the aortic arch out of the free end of the graft. Once this process is complete the graft is clamped distal to the side arm so the bypass, including the cerebral perfusion, is recommenced. The descending thoracic aorta is clamped so that the distal perfusion can be commenced. A small clamp is placed on the subclavian artery (Fig. 6.8f). The distal anastomosis is performed between the dacron graft and the descending thoracic aorta with the monofilament suture (Fig. 6.8g). Once completed, the two aortic clamps are released.

After the rewarming is complete, cardiopulmonary bypass is discontinued and the 8 mm graft is anastomosed to the origin of the subclavian artery (Fig. 6.8h).

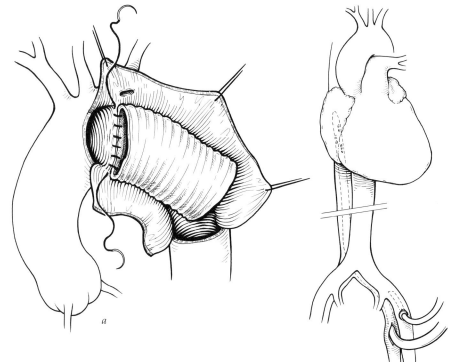

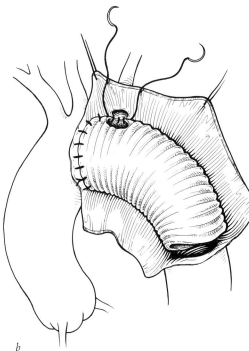

Fig. 6.8
Distal arch aneurysm repair with deep hypothermic circulatory arrest.

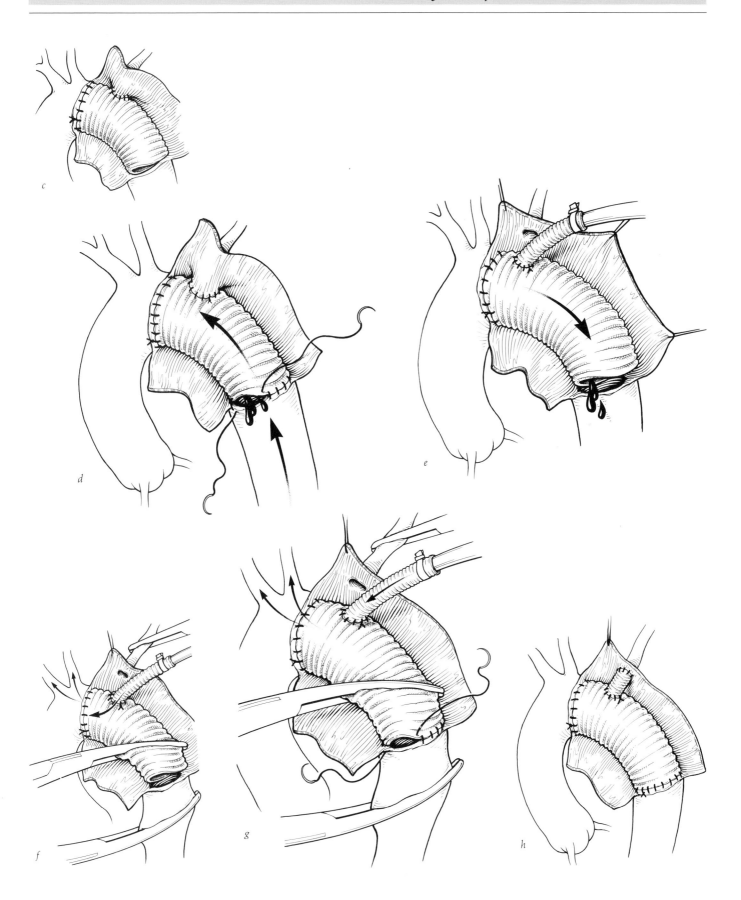

DESCENDING THORACIC AORTIC ANEURYSMS

Repair with tube graft

Elective surgery is usually indicated on aneurysms of the descending thoracic aorta when they reach a maximum transverse diameter of 6–7 cm. Semi-urgent indications for operation include the presence of back pain, pressure on the vertebral column or chest wall, the development of hoarseness from recurrent laryngeal nerve palsy or compression of the left main bronchus. Leakage of the aneurysm into the left pleural cavity or frank rupture are life-threatening emergencies.

Adequate exposure of the descending thoracic aorta is essential. The proximal end is usually approached through an incision in the fourth intercostal space extending from the neck of the rib posteriorly to the anterior end of the intercostal space. Further exposure can be obtained by dividing the neck of the fifth rib posteriorly. For aneurysms extending inferiorly, the sixth and seventh space is more satisfactory with removal of the anterior end of the sixth rib and crossing the costal margin if necessary. Very extensive aneurysms of the descending thoracic aorta may be approached using a bucket handle technique where the upper end is approached through the fourth intercostal space and the lower end anastomosed through the seventh or eighth intercostal space. Thoracoabdominal aneurysms are approached using the sixth intercostal space, extending the incision through the costal margin into the retroperitoneal space and extending for a variable distance vertically, depending on the pathology. While some surgeons prefer to repair these aneurysms using a simple cross-clamp technique, our preference is to use left heart bypass from the left atrium to the femoral artery (Fig. 5.9). Partial cardiopulmonary bypass is also satisfactory using a left-sided femoral vein to femoral artery bypass (Fig. 5.10).

The aneurysm is exposed by lifting the lung forward, dividing any adhesions. The phrenic and vagus nerves together with the recurrent laryngeal branch are identified and mobilized if necessary. The pleura is opened and the aneurysm neck encircled with a tape. Similarly, the pleura is opened inferiorly at the lower extent of the aneurysm and the aorta encircled with a tape. It is important at this stage to avoid digital dissection and this should be performed with a curved clamp to avoid avulsion of the intercostal arteries, which can cause troublesome bleeding from a relatively inaccessible site. Left atriofemoral bypass is commenced and, when the circulation is stable, the aorta is clamped proximally and distally to isolate the aneurysm. A longitudinal incision is made in the lateral wall of the aneurysm sac and a small transverse incision made at each end of the incision (Fig. 6.9a). The intercostal arteries are identified. Intercostal arteries should be preserved when the aneurysm extends distally, when the intercostal vessels are large and particularly when large intercostal vessels have a relatively poor back-flow. In most cases of descending thoracic aortic aneurysms involving the upper part of the descending thoracic aorta, no attempt is made to save these vessels, which are oversewn. The surgical techniques to identify the important intercostal arteries are discussed above (see Chapter 5, pp.50–51).

Once all intercostal bleeding is controlled, a dacron graft is then chosen to match the diameter of the thoracic aorta. The proximal suture line commences laterally and then continues posteriorly (Fig. 6.9b); suturing of the anterior wall completes the anastomosis.

A clamp is placed on the dacron graft and the proximal aortic clamp released gently to check the haemostasis at the suture line. Additional sutures may be placed at this time. Once haemostasis has been achieved, attention is turned to the lower end. The graft is stretched or alternatively a clamp is placed distally and the graft is allowed to fill and expand so that the level of the lower anastomosis can be gauged accurately. The clamp is then placed proximally and the lower end of the graft divided for the lower anastomosis. The anastomosis is performed with a continuous monofilament suture (Fig. 6.9c). Prior to closure of the lower end of the anterior wall the distal clamp is released to ensure that there is no embolic material. Similarly, the proximal clamp on the dacron graft is released gradually. The anastomosis is completed and a small needle is placed in the dacron graft to ensure that there is no air left in the graft (Fig. 6.9d). The left heart bypass is then discontinued and the lower clamp released first. The proximal clamp is released very slowly over a period of minutes, during which time the patient's circulation and biochemical parameters are monitored.

The upper and lower suture lines and the intercostal arteries in the aneurysm sac are inspected. Once the haemostasis is completed the sac is closed loosely over the graft.

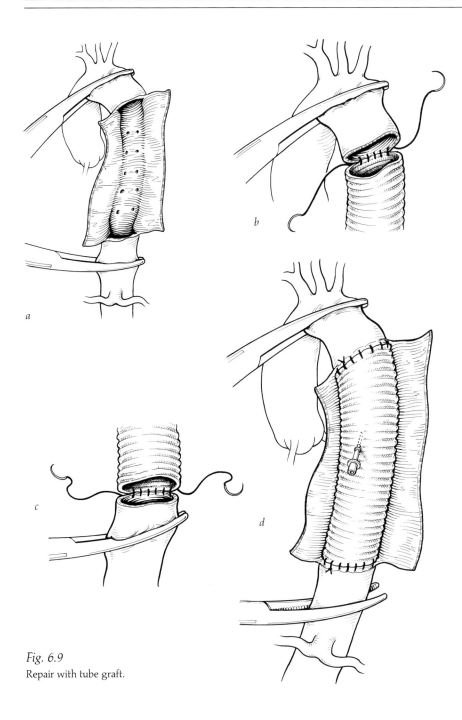

Special problems

When mobilizing an aneurysm of the distal third of the aorta, care must be taken to avoid damage to the oesophagus or the lung. Dissection of the upper end of the aneurysm can result in damage to the phrenic, the vagus and recurrent nerve. Every effort should be made to identify and protect these structures.

The sequence of flushing, de-airing and unclamping is of paramount importance so that embolic or particulate matter is avoided and the flow from the distal aorta is not directed proximally during unclamping the aorta.

Fig. 6.9
Repair with tube graft.

Elephant trunk: stage II

The second stage of the elephant trunk procedure is performed through a left posterolateral thoracotomy or thoracoabdominal incision according to the length of descending thoracic or thoracoabdominal aneurysm.

Control of the upper descending thoracic aorta is facilitated by the presence of thrombus around the redundant 'elephant trunk' graft. This is achieved through a small incision in the upper descending thoracic aorta distal to the old suture line and left subclavian artery (Fig. 6.10a). (This does not bleed because of the presence of thrombus in this region.) The index finger is inserted around the dacron graft between the graft and the aortic wall through the area of thrombus. The terminal end of the dacron graft is lifted out through the aortic incision, controlled between the index finger and thumb until an aortic clamp is applied (Fig. 6.10b). The aortic incision is then lengthened and an additional segment of dacron graft is anastomosed to the end of the 'elephant trunk'. The distal reconstruction between the thoracic aorta and thoracoabdominal aorta depends on the distal extent of the aneurysm.

Traumatic rupture of the thoracic aorta

Blunt trauma to the chest or abdomen can cause rupture of the aorta (Passaro & Pace 1959). The descending thoracic aorta just beyond the subclavian artery in the region of the isthmus is the most commonly affected site. Relative frequencies are shown in Figure 6.11a. Traumatic rupture of the thoracic aorta is commonly associated with other potentially lethal injuries and therefore a complete assessment of the patient is essential.

The diagnosis can be suspected on the chest X-ray and confirmed on CT scan or transoesophageal echocardiography. The definitive diagnosis still requires digital subtraction angiography. A persisting Kommeral diverticulum can mimic a localized traumatic rupture of the isthmus.

Surgical exposure of the upper descending thoracic aorta is through a posterolateral thoracotomy using the fourth interspace. Some surgeons prefer simple aortic cross-clamping of the aorta above and below the site of rupture. However, our preference is to use left heart bypass or femorofemoral bypass to secure more stable operating conditions. Heparin-coated tubing avoids the need for systemic heparin, which may be contraindicated by the presence of central nervous system or abdominal injuries. Although uncommon, repair of a rupture involving the aortic arch requires the use of deep hypothermic circulatory arrest.

Proximal control of the aorta above the site of the rupture can be difficult in patients with acute traumatic rupture. The haematoma is often confined only by the outer layer of the adventitia and it is necessary to dissect well proximal to the site of the rupture to obtain normal aortic wall for clamping and to avoid entering the haematoma. Mobilization of the vagus nerve and recurrent laryngeal nerve may be required to provide access to the distal aortic arch (Fig. 6.11b). In some patients, it is necessary to clamp between the left subclavian and left common carotid arteries to obtain sufficient length of proximal aorta. In an emergency, proximal control can be obtained by passing a finger superiorly between the left subclavian and left common carotid arteries prior to clamping (Turney & Rodriguez 1990) (Fig. 6.11c, d).

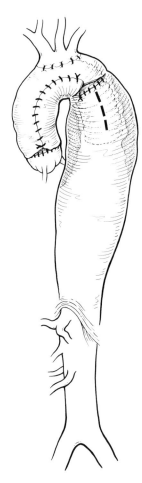
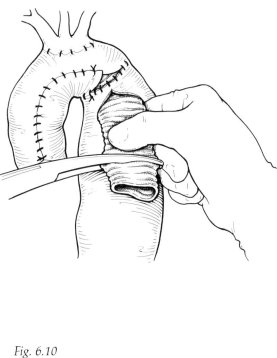

Fig. 6.10
Elephant trunk procedure: stage II.

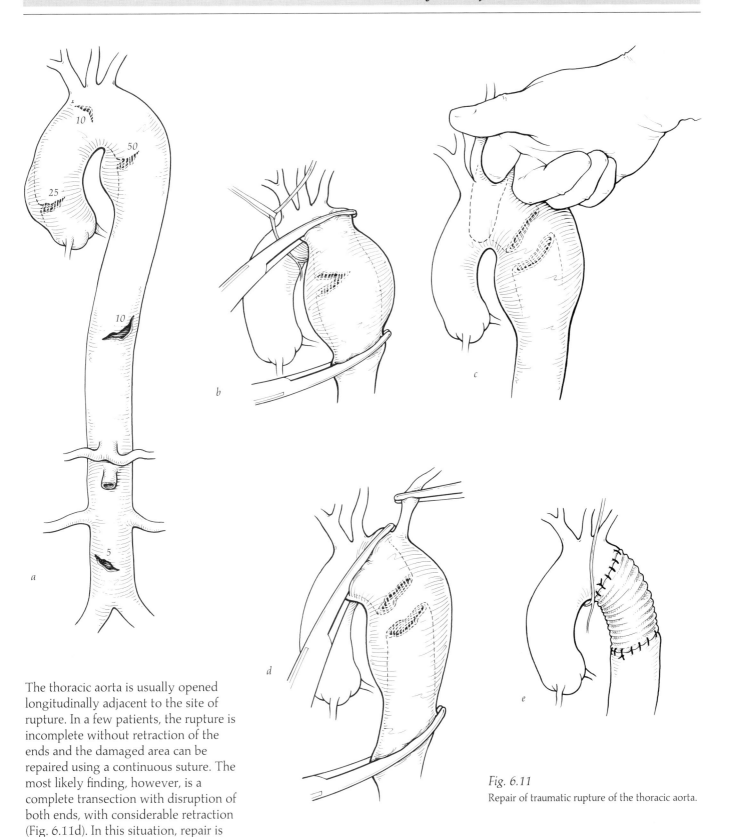

The thoracic aorta is usually opened longitudinally adjacent to the site of rupture. In a few patients, the rupture is incomplete without retraction of the ends and the damaged area can be repaired using a continuous suture. The most likely finding, however, is a complete transection with disruption of both ends, with considerable retraction (Fig. 6.11d). In this situation, repair is usually performed using a short interposition graft (Fig. 6.11e).

Fig. 6.11
Repair of traumatic rupture of the thoracic aorta.

Acute traumatic rupture of the aorta frequently occurs in young patients who have no pre-existing aortic disease and in whom there is no collateral blood supply to the spinal cord predisposing to paraplegia. The use of cardiopulmonary bypass, avoidance of hypovolaemia and the ligation of the minimum number of intercostal vessels will minimize the risk of paraplegia.

Chronic traumatic rupture

Finding a calcified aneurysm in an otherwise healthy patient who has a past history of major thoracic or abdominal trauma is an infrequent but increasingly common finding. The natural history of chronic post-traumatic rupture of the thoracic aorta is one of progressive enlargement which may lead to rupture. Surgical repair is recommended in these aneurysms unless there is a contraindication (Zehnder 1956).

The approach is similar to that of an acute traumatic rupture except, when the aneurysm is large, access to the upper end may be more difficult. Unlike an atherosclerotic aneurysm, the proximal and distal aorta is relatively normal and left heart bypass or femorofemoral bypass will usually suffice. It is rarely necessary to use deep hypothermia and circulatory arrest under these circumstances.

The surgical procedure is similar to acute rupture, except that it is necessary to replace the site of chronic traumatic rupture with a short interposition dacron graft.

False aneurysms following aortic surgery

False aneurysms are often the result of poor surgical technique. Use of the graft inclusion technique at the initial operation may put excessive tension on coronary artery suture lines. If bleeding occurs within the aneurysm sac, which has been closed tightly over the graft, partial dehiscence and/or false aneurysm formation may result (Kouchoukos et al 1986). Second procedures on the aorta are always difficult and every attempt should be made to prevent suture line dehiscence.

REFERENCES

Bentall H, De Bono A 1968 A technique for complete replacement of the ascending aorta. Thorax 23: 338–339
Borst H G 1981 Replacement of ascending aorta and aortic valve. Annals of Thoracic Surgery 32: 613–614
Borst H G, Schaudig A, Rudolph W 1964 Arteriovenous fistula of the aortic arch: repair during deep hypothermia and circulatory arrest. Journal of Thoracic and Cardiovascular Surgery 48: 443–447
Cabrol C, Pavie A, Gandjbakhch I et al 1981 Complete replacement of the ascending aorta with reimplantation of the coronary arteries: new surgical approach. Journal of Thoracic and Cardiovascular Surgery 81: 309–315
Crawford E S, Svensson L G, Coselli J S, Safi H J, Hess K R 1989 Surgical treatment of aneurysm and/or dissection of the ascending aorta, transverse aortic arch, and ascending aorta and transverse aortic arch: factors influencing survival in 717 patients. Journal of Thoracic and Cardiovascular Surgery 98: 659–674
Kouchoukos N T 1991 Composite graft replacement of the ascending aorta and aortic valve with the inclusion-wrap and open techniques. Seminars in Thoracic and Cardiovascular Surgery 3: 171–176
Kouchoukos N T, Marshall W G Jr, Wedige-Stecher T A 1986 Eleven-year experience with composite graft replacement of the ascending aorta and aortic valve. Journal of Thoracic and Cardiovascular Surgery 92: 691–705

Liversay J J, Cooley D A, Duncan J M, Ott D A, Walker W E, Reul G J 1982 Open aortic anastomosis: improved results in the treatment of aneurysms of the aortic arch. Circulation 66 (suppl I): 122–126
Matalanis G, Buxton B 1993 Retrograde vital organ perfusion during aortic arch repair. Annals of Thoracic Surgery 56: 981–984
Passaro E Jr, Pace W G 1959 Traumatic rupture of the aorta. Surgery 46: 787–791
Turney S Z, Rodriguez A 1990 Injuries to the great thoracic vessels. In: Turney S Z, Rodriguez A, Cowley R D (eds) Management of cardiothoracic trauma. Williams & Wilkins, Baltimore, pp 229–260
Wheat M W Jr, Wilson J R, Bartley T D 1964 Successful replacement of the entire ascending aorta and aortic valve. Journal of the American Medical Association 188: 717–719
Zehnder M A 1956 Delayed post-traumatic rupture of the aorta in a young healthy individual after closed injury: mechanical–etiological considerations. Angiology 7: 252–267
Zubiate P, Kay J H 1976 Surgical treatment of aneurysm of the ascending aorta with aortic sufficiency and marked displacement of the coronary ostia. Journal of Thoracic and Cardiovascular Surgery 71: 415–421

Chapter 7

Aortic dissections and dissecting aneurysms

Brian Buxton   **George Matalanis**

DISSECTION OF THE THORACIC AORTA

The surgical management of an aortic dissection is frequently more complicated than that of a simple aortic aneurysm. The catastrophic presentation with rupture into the pericardium causing tamponade or into the pleural cavity and with obstruction of the major arterial branches may lead to a complex surgical problem which requires an early diagnosis and specialized surgical techniques to achieve a satisfactory result. Aortic dissections are classified as acute if they present to the surgeon less than 2 weeks from the time of the first symptoms or chronic if appearing later.

The Stanford anatomic classification of aortic dissection is now widely accepted and forms the basis for the treatment strategy (Daily et al 1970). The classification is based on whether or not the ascending thoracic aorta is involved and it is not dependent on the site of origin (Fig. 7.1a). Type A dissections involve the ascending thoracic aorta and also may involve the arch or descending thoracic aorta. Type B dissections do not involve the ascending thoracic aorta and most are confined to the descending thoracic aorta but sometimes involve the arch. Type A dissections commonly rupture into the pericardium causing cardiac tamponade and are sometimes associated with aortic regurgitation and coronary artery occlusion. Type B dissections rupture less frequently than type A dissections but, when rupture occurs, it is usually into the pleural cavity, often with exsanguination. Major aortic branch occlusion occurs with either type A or type B dissections. Type A dissections are associated with a very poor prognosis: 80% of patients are dead in 2 weeks, mostly through rupture into the pericardium. On the other hand, type B dissections are more benign and 70% survive to become chronic (Hirst 1958).

Investigations

Investigations are often required urgently, particularly in type A dissections. Transoesophageal Doppler echocardiography can be performed rapidly and will normally confirm the presence and location of a dissection. It will also provide information about the site of origin and whether or not there is cardiac tamponade or aortic regurgitation and is therefore almost ideal when the presentation is acute (Erbel et al 1989, Hashimoto et al 1989). Dynamic computed tomography scanning, magnetic resonance imaging and conventional angiography will provide additional information but are more time consuming.

Indications for operation

Surgery is indicated in most acute type A dissections. Patients with coma or with bowel necrosis are the exception and need to be evaluated carefully before embarking on surgery. Type B dissections, on the other hand, are treated medically unless there is evidence of continued pain, rupture or branch occlusion. The type of operation depends on the aetiology of the dissection, duration of the symptoms, a detailed knowledge of the site of origin and extension of the dissection, the state of the aortic valve, and anatomy of the coronary arteries and other major aortic branches.

Surgical management

The detailed surgical management differs from the management of simple aortic aneurysms in that the aorta is not only dissected but is very friable, and to prevent a secondary injury the use of aortic clamps is avoided where possible (Livesay et al 1982, Cooley 1991) (Fig. 7.1b, c). The suture lines require additional reinforcement to prevent excessive haemorrhage and to minimize the chance of residual dissection. Cardiopulmonary bypass can be complicated by the presence of the false channel which may supply some of the major aortic vessels. Because major vessels may be supplied by the false channel in chronic dissections, the branch anatomy should be defined prior to surgery.

Special considerations in chronic dissection

While in acute dissections it is desirable to obliterate the false channel completely, this may be disadvantageous in the chronic phase. With the passage of time after the dissection, the blood supply to some important aortic branches (e.g. carotid, renal, visceral and spinal) becomes entirely dependent on flow in the false channel. Thus, obliteration of the false channel may result in acute ischaemia in those territories. Furthermore, the true lumen tends to become narrow and cannot be re-expanded to appose the outer wall of the false channel, even in the non-aneurysmal segments.

For these reasons we prefer to 'fenestrate' the remaining dissected aorta at the site of the distal anastomosis to the graft. This consists of a local resection in the form of a 'D' of the wall between the true and false channels at the site of the distal anastomosis. The anastomosis is thus performed to the false channel wall over about two-thirds of the circumference of the aorta. While this may seem unappealing on the grounds that continued perfusion of the false channel may accelerate false aneurysm formation, it is a reasonable compromise. The alternative would entail resection of undilated dissected aorta and individual branch vessel re-attachment, with attendant higher morbidity and mortality.

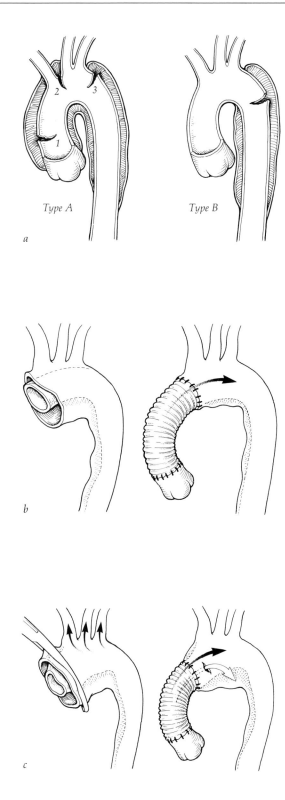

TYPE A DISSECTIONS

Repair of dissection of ascending thoracic aorta with tube graft under deep hypothermic circulatory arrest

This procedure is usually performed urgently once the diagnosis of type A dissection has been confirmed. Tube graft replacement of the ascending thoracic aorta is indicated in those patients who have no evidence of a connective tissue disorder such as Marfan's disease or cystic medial necrosis, and the coronary artery and aortic valve anatomy are normal. The procedure should be avoided in patients with connective tissue disorders because of the possibility of developing dilatation of the aortic root proximal to the tube graft.

The approach is via a median sternotomy using deep hypothermic circulatory arrest, unless the dissection is very localized. The procedure is performed by cannulating the femoral artery and femoral vein which can, if necessary, be performed under local anaesthesia to obtain vascular access and control. If the dissection has continued distally, care should be taken to avoid cannulating the false channel in the femoral artery cannulation. A vent is then placed in the right superior pulmonary vein and passed through the left atrium into the left ventricle. A catheter is introduced into the coronary sinus for retrograde cardioplegia and a separate cannula placed in the superior vena cava for retrograde cerebral perfusion (Fig. 5.7).

The operation is performed using deep hypothermia and circulatory arrest (see Ch. 5, p. 46).

Fig. 7.1

(a) Stanford classification of aortic dissection.
(b) Open repair of dissection.
(c) Closed repair of dissection.

The aorta is opened widely on the anterior surface. The intimal flap is trimmed and the aorta is partially or completely transected above and below (Fig. 7.2b). The upper and lower suture lines are reinforced by glycerol resorcinol formaldehyde (GRF) glue (Fig. 7.2c). The GRF is a two-part glue in which the glycerol resorcinol component is polymerized by the addition of formaldehyde. The glue can only be used on dry surfaces and is washed away and fails to solidify in the presence of blood. The glycerol resorcinol component is placed between the dissected layers of the aorta extending for approximately 2–3 cm. Prior to insertion, the glue is warmed to between 40°C and 50°C. One or two drops of formaldehyde solution are placed directly on the glue through a small 25 gauge needle to commence the hardening process. During activation of the glue, it is important to compress both layers of the aorta to promote adhesion between the layers of the dissection. Blood can be kept away during deep hypothermia by turning off the retrograde circulation and by compressing the layers with the use of a large Foley balloon catheter (Fig. 7.2d). Alternatively, the glue can be inserted and the layers of the dissection oversewn and compressed with a cotton sponge (see Fig. 7.3e). If the GRF glue is not available, a teflon strip can be inserted between the dissected layers and the dissection oversewn (Fig. 7.2f). A graft is selected to match the diameter of the aorta. This graft is cut, obliquely if necessary, to match the distal aorta. The distal anastomosis is performed first, commencing at the left side and passing along a posterior wall (Fig. 6.4b). The anastomosis is completed along the anterior wall (Fig. 7.2e). Cardiopulmonary bypass is then recommenced, flushing any particulate material through the aortic graft (Fig. 6.4c). The cerebral perfusion is discontinued and a clamp is placed on the dacron graft proximal to the distal

anastomosis (Figs 7.2g and 6.4d). Cardiopulmonary bypass pump flow is increased to normal and the patient rewarmed. The graft is placed under tension and transected at the level of the proposed proximal suture line. The proximal anastomosis is performed with a monofilament suture, commencing to the left and passing posteriorly above the left coronary artery orifice. The anastomosis is completed passing anteriorly to the right. Prior to completion of the proximal anastomosis, the left ventricular vent is stopped, the heart filled with blood and any air evacuated. The suture is then tied and a vent placed in the dacron graft to continue the removal of air (Fig. 7.2g). The clamp is removed from the dacron graft to allow the blood to enter the coronary circulation.

Rewarming is continued until the rectal temperature reaches 38°C. Haemostasis is checked and the sac closed over the dacron graft.

In the presence of a very localized dissection of the ascending thoracic aorta, deep hypothermic circulatory arrest is avoided if the clamp can be placed in the distal ascending thoracic aorta. The surgical technique is similar to the preceding except that the patient's temperature is lowered to about 30°C and the aorta cross-clamped proximal to the innominate artery. The aneurysm sac is opened and transected above and below. The layers of the dissection are repaired either with a teflon sandwich or the GRF glue. The sequence of aortic anastomoses is then reversed, with a proximal anastomosis being performed first and the distal anastomosis last. After removal of air from the heart and ascending thoracic aorta, the aortic clamp is released. All bleeding points are secured and the aneurysm sac is loosely wrapped over the anterior surface of the dacron graft.

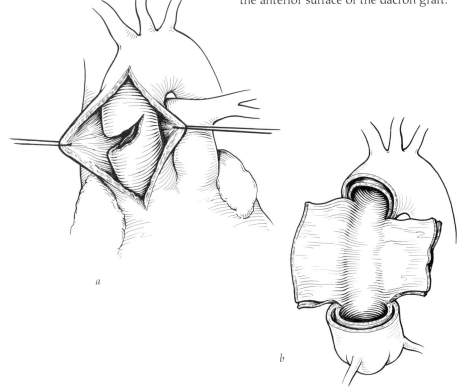

a

b

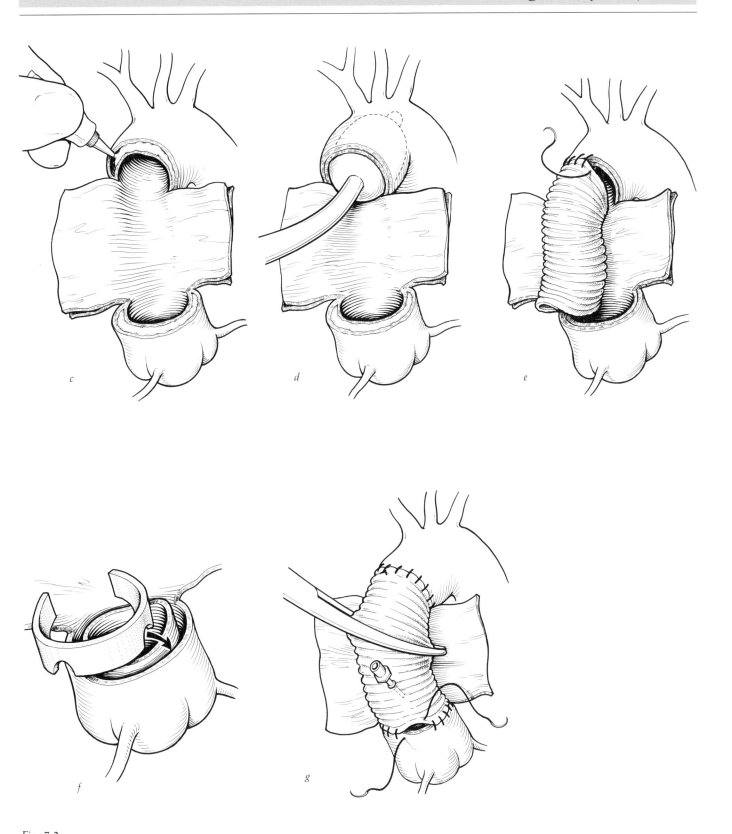

Fig. 7.2

Repair of dissection of ascending thoracic aorta with tube graft under deep hypothermic circulatory arrest.

Ascending aortic dissection with aortic valve involvement

Aortic valve repair

Every attempt should be made to repair the aortic valve in patients with aortic dissection. Aortic valve repair is contraindicated in patients with a connective tissue disorder such as annuloaortic ectasia or Marfan's disease, where progressive dilatation of the aortic root is very likely to result in recurrence of the aortic regurgitation. Detachment of the inner layer of the aorta in the region of the aortic valve commonly results in the loss of commissural support of the valve leaflets, which prolapse into the ventricular cavity, resulting in aortic regurgitation (Fig. 7.3a). Aortic dissection rarely damages the aortic valve leaflets, so that normal valve function can usually be restored.

Repair of the aortic valve under these circumstances is relatively simple and consists of resuspension of the valve commissure or commissures by means of teflon pledgets and obliteration of the dissection space either with GRF glue or the use of intramural teflon. If there is dissection into the aortic root, the orifices of the coronary arteries may be involved and they should be inspected carefully at the time of aortic valve repair.

The repair is performed prior to performing the proximal anastomosis. GRF glue is placed in the wall of the aorta and polymerized by the formaldehyde solution. A suture supported by teflon pledgets (on the inside and outside of the aorta) is placed at the upper limit of the commissure, which is resuspended to the aortic wall in the normal or a slightly higher position (Fig. 7.3b, c). A buttress suture each side of the commissure on either side may give stronger support (Fig. 7.3d). The layers of the dissection are then closed with a continuous

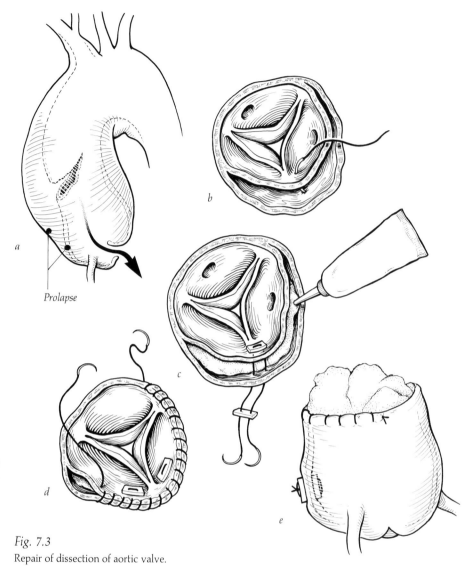

Fig. 7.3
Repair of dissection of aortic valve.

suture. A gauze swab is placed in the aortic root to balloon the coronary sinuses and attach the inner and outer layers of the dissected aortic root (Fig. 7.3e). This process normally takes 10–15 minutes. The aortic graft is then anastomosed to the repaired aortic root with a monofilament suture.

Valve repair is successful in about 80% of patients who have an aortic dissection with loss of commissure support and leaflet prolapse. The aortic valve should not be repaired in patients with connective tissue disorder or annular dilatation because this will almost certainly result in recurrence and the necessity for reoperation. In about 20% of patients, valve repair is not possible and aortic valve replacement should be performed.

Aortic valve replacement

Aortic valve replacement (as part of a valve conduit) should be performed in all patients with connective tissue disorder, aortic root disease or aortic regurgitation due to annular dilatation. Isolated aortic valve replacement may be performed in some patients with aortic regurgitation and dissection without a connective tissue disorder. Aortic valve replacement under these circumstances is usually straightforward and is performed after repair of the dissection in the proximal aorta (Fig. 7.4a, b). The preference is for intra-annular valve implantation with supra-aortic valve pledgets (Fig. 7.4c, d). This technique, however, may result in lateral displacement of the coronary artery orifice. If the pledgets are too close to the coronary orifice, implantation of the coronary artery orifices into the graft becomes more difficult (Fig. 7.4e).

The technique of supra-annular valve replacement with subannular pledgets is an alternative (Fig. 7.4f) and is a very strong technique. When used in conjunction with a valve conduit, this technique facilitates the implantation of the coronary artery orifices into the side of the dacron conduit.

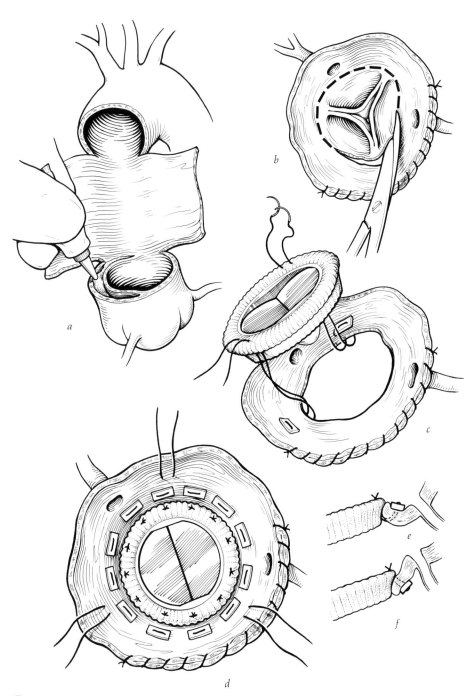

Fig. 7.4
Aortic valve replacement.

Coronary artery dissection

Minor dissection of a coronary artery can be repaired directly by reconstitution of the aortic wall around the dissected coronary artery (Fig. 7.5a, b). A more extensive disruption of the coronary artery orifices, for example when the intimal tear extends into the orifice of the coronary artery itself, is probably better repaired indirectly using a bypass graft rather than attempting a difficult repair of the orifice which might result in stenosis or occlusion.

Coronary artery repair
Direct repair of a minor coronary dissection is performed after confirming the patency of the coronary artery orifice by the passage of a 2 mm or 2.5 mm dilator (Fig. 7.5c). The aortic root is repaired around the coronary artery by use of the GRF glue technique and oversewing the dissection (Fig. 7.5c, d). Again, the aortic root is distended with the use of a gauze swab or Fogarty catheter to compress the two layers during the polymerization of the glue (Fig. 7.3e). Alternatively, the teflon sandwich technique can be used with satisfactory results (Fig. 7.2f).

Coronary artery bypass
Coronary artery bypass should be used where there is any doubt about the patency of the main coronary artery (Fig. 7.5e). An internal mammary artery or a saphenous vein graft is anastomosed distally during the period of cardiac standstill. The proximal end is then anastomosed to the side of the dacron graft after a small window has been created by electrocautery (Fig. 7.5f).

An internal mammary artery bypass graft is preferable to a saphenous vein graft reconstruction in younger patients because of the superior late patency. If grafted to the left system, an internal mammary graft has the additional advantage of not requiring a proximal anastomosis (Fig. 7.5f).

Coexisting coronary artery disease

Coronary artery disease is not infrequently found in patients with a chronic aortic dissection. Repair of coronary artery stenoses should be considered during repair of a chronic dissection and even during the repair of an acute dissection if the coronary anatomy has been defined.

Distal anastomoses are performed between the saphenous vein and/or the internal mammary artery grafts and the native coronary circulation. The proximal ends of the saphenous vein grafts are attached to the dacron graft after excision of a small ellipse of tissue from the anterior surface of the dacron graft using electrocautery. The anastomoses are usually performed using a 5/0 monofilament suture. The aneurysm sac is repaired around the coronary artery bypass grafts after excision of small scallops from the cut edge of the aneurysm sac.

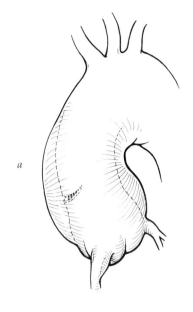

a

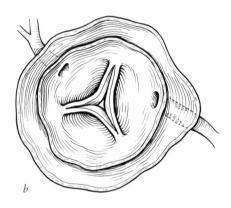

b

Fig. 7.5
Repair of coronary artery dissection.

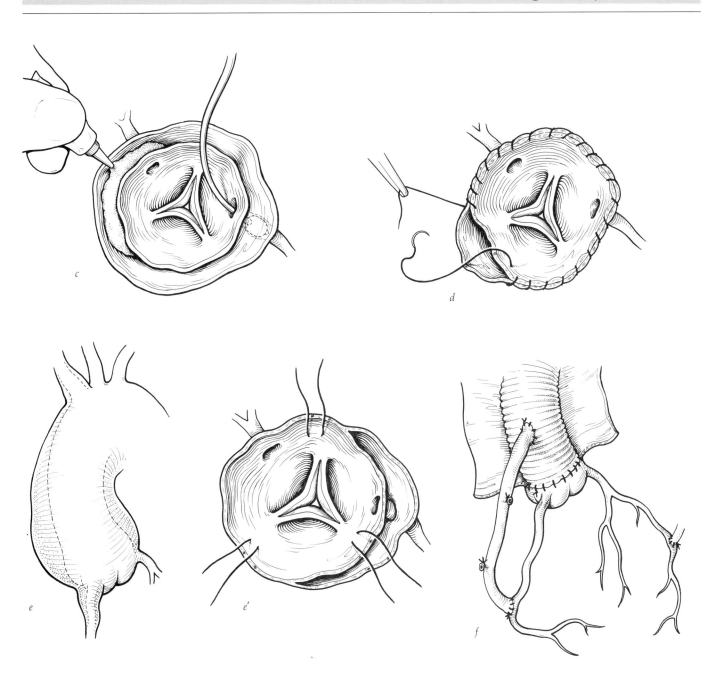

Dissection of the aortic root and ascending thoracic aorta

A composite valve conduit is used in patients who have a dissection of the aortic root complicated by aortic regurgitation in whom the valve cannot be repaired, and in all patients who have aortic root disease associated with a connective tissue disorder. The aortic valve and ascending thoracic aorta can be replaced separately, leaving aortic root tissue around the coronary arteries if the aortic root is normal.

The aortic valve conduit technique
This operation is performed through a median sternotomy, usually with deep hypothermic circulatory arrest to avoid the use of clamps on the distal ascending thoracic aorta (Figs 5.6–5.8).

With the head down, the aorta is opened longitudinally to display the inner layer of the dissection and intimal tears. The aorta is transected just proximal to the innominate artery and the layers repaired with GRF glue or a teflon felt inlay (Fig. 7.2c, d). A graft is sutured end to end to the distal aorta with a running prolene suture (Fig. 7.2e). The bypass is recommenced, and after all embolic material has been flushed from the graft (Fig. 6.4c) and from the cerebral vessels, the graft is clamped and the retrograde cerebral perfusion is ceased. Cardiopulmonary bypass is recommenced (Fig. 7.6a).

The aortic root is transected above the level of the coronary arteries. The aortic valve is excised, the aortic diameter measured and a dacron valve conduit is sutured into the annulus with interrupted dacron sutures with teflon pledgets.

The left coronary artery orifice is circumscribed with a 3–4 mm rim of aortic wall (Fig. 6.3f, g). The coronary artery is mobilized for about 1 cm so that it can be anastomosed without tension to the graft. A small ellipse of dacron is excised from the wall of the graft adjacent to the coronary artery (Fig. 7.6b), to which the latter is anastomosed with a running suture. The graft is then lifted towards the head and the right coronary artery is mobilized with a button of tissue and anastomosed to the side of the graft in a similar fashion.

The conduit containing the valve and the aortic graft is then transected and sutured to the distal ascending thoracic graft with a running monofilament suture (Fig. 7.6c). Prior to completion of the suture line, the heart is filled with blood and air evacuated from the aortic root. A needle is placed in the ascending thoracic aortic graft and the aortic clamp released. The sac is wrapped around the graft.

Localized dissection of the aortic root
If dissection is confined to the ascending thoracic aorta, or if the distal ascending thoracic aorta appears to be of good quality, it is possible to replace the aortic root by clamping the distal ascending thoracic aorta and using a normal cardiopulmonary bypass technique.

In this operation, the sequence is usually reversed. The aortic valve and conduit are implanted into the annulus first, the left and then the right coronary anastomoses and finally the distal anastomosis are performed between the repaired aorta and the distal end of the valve conduit.

The Cabrol technique with a separate coronary artery to dacron graft (Cabrol et al 1981)
This technique is suited to patients with an aneurysm or dissection of the aorta in whom a valve conduit is indicated but in whom the coronary artery orifices are relatively low, making direct implantation difficult (Cabrol et al 1986). The operation is done either under deep hypothermic circulatory arrest or with normal bypass circuit, depending on the distal extent of the dissection.

The aorta is opened longitudinally and the pathology defined. After excision of the aortic valve, a separate 8 mm dacron graft is anastomosed directly to the left coronary artery orifice (Fig. 7.7a). The valve conduit is selected to match the size of the aortic root and sutured into the aortic annulus with braided dacron sutures and teflon pledgets (Fig. 7.7b). The 8 mm dacron graft is then brought posteriorly and is anastomosed to the right coronary artery orifice (Fig. 7.7c).

An oval window of dacron is created in the side of the conduit and a side-to-side anastomosis is then performed between the 8 mm coronary conduit and the main aortic graft (Fig. 7.7c). It is important to avoid kinking the 8 mm graft between the aortic and right coronary anastomosis by correct positioning of the side-to-side anastomosis with the aorta (Fig. 7.7d). The reconstruction is completed by anastomosing the main graft to the distal ascending thoracic aorta. A particular difficulty with this technique is the tendency of the 8 mm graft to angulate between the right coronary artery orifice anastomosis and the side-to-side anastomosis. Decompression of the false sac by suturing into the right atrial appendage is usually not necessary as haemostasis can be achieved readily because of the good exposure.

Another theoretical problem is that the coronary circulation is dependent on a short interposition of dacron graft between the main graft and the coronary artery orifice, and this may pose an additional risk to long-term coronary artery patency.

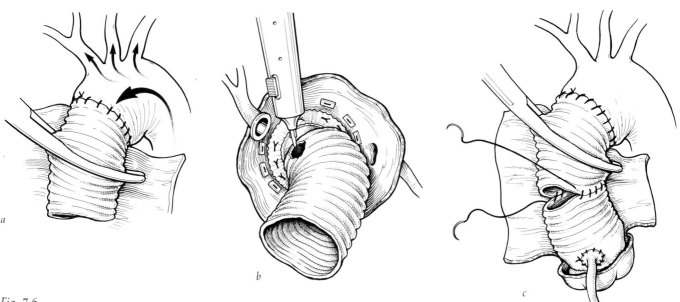

Fig. 7.6
Dissection of aortic root and ascending thoracic aorta with valve conduit.

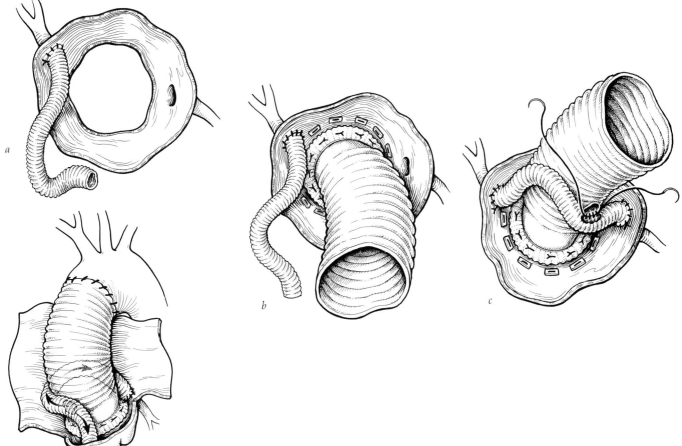

Fig. 7.7
Cabrol technique.

Post-traumatic dissection

Post-traumatic dissection can occur as the result of blunt trauma with partial rupture of the upper descending thoracic aorta, ascending thoracic aorta or the aortic arch. In survivors, localized dissection is a common finding (Fig. 7.8a). The surgical management of these patients is described under post-traumatic rupture (see Ch. 6).

Post-surgical dissection

With the advent of cardiac surgery, post-surgical dissections are becoming more frequent. Over-zealous application of the partial occlusion clamp can cause dissection of the ascending thoracic aorta (Fig. 7.8b). Failure to suture the full thickness of the aorta with a proximal coronary artery anastomosis can also lead to dissection of the ascending thoracic aorta. The aortic cannulation site and the aortic cardioplegia needle sites can also initiate a traumatic dissection (Fig. 7.8c).

Residual dissections of the distal ascending thoracic aorta, arch and descending thoracic aorta are relatively common following repair of a proximal dissection and do not necessarily require repair. Increasing symptoms or progressive enlargement of the false sac may be an indication for reoperation. A surgical dissection of the ascending thoracic aorta may present intraoperatively or after surgery. The surgical techniques used to repair the dissection are outlined in other sections. However, the approach differs depending on when the dissection occurs.

Intraoperative aortic dissection

Dissection from aortic clamp, cannulation site or suture line can be a catastrophic event and needs to be dealt with immediately and effectively if the patient is to survive.

Relocation of the arterial cannula is necessary to provide access for the repair. The cannula is usually transferred from the aorta to the common femoral artery on the right side so that the repair can be performed under deep hypothermia with wide access to the proximal aorta.

Once the appropriate temperature has been reached and the bypass discontinued, the dissection site is explored and repaired either with GRF glue or the use of teflon strips. Resection and replacement grafting is rarely required.

Acute postoperative dissection

Acute dissection during cardiac surgery sometimes goes unrecognized at the initial operation and may present in the first 2 weeks following cardiac surgery. Progressive enlargement of the aorta, cardiac tamponade and branch obstruction are common presentations which usually require immediate repair.

Re-entry into the chest is usually not difficult in the first 2 weeks following the initial operation. Cannulation of the right common femoral artery and femoral vein, however, add a degree of safety and facilitate the repair, which can be supplemented, if necessary, by deep hypothermic circulatory arrest.

Residual dissection

Residual dissection may follow a previous repair of aortic dissection in which the false sac is not obliterated and continues to fill from the aortic suture line or from a re-entry site more distally (Crawford et al 1984). Regular follow-up of patients after repair of the aortic dissection is therefore essential to detect new areas of dilation and potential rupture (Miller 1991).

Late repair of post-surgical dissections

Reoperation can be particularly difficult if there is enlargement of the dissection sac anteriorly. Femoral cannulation, full cardiopulmonary bypass and even deep hypothermic circulatory arrest may be required to minimize the risks of uncontrolled haemorrhage during the sternotomy.

To reopen the sternum following a previous operation, the midline incision is usually carried further inferiorly towards the umbilicus and a 5–7 cm incision made in the upper linea alba. The edges of the linea alba are then elevated in the space behind the sternum (Fig. 7.8d) and the xiphisternal attachments of the diaphragm divided laterally to display the pericardium and the anterior wall of the right ventricle. The dissection is performed with long scissors with the sternum elevated using retractors, and the dissection carried out under direct vision (Fig. 7.8e).

Intravenous nitroglycerine and elevation of the patient's head will help lower the right-sided pressures and avoid damage to the right ventricle. If the aneurysm sac is adherent to the posterior wall of the sternum, it is difficult to avoid injury, particularly if the sac is thin walled. Deep hypothermia associated with reduced cardiopulmonary bypass flows or even circulatory arrest may be essential if the aneurysm sac is opened inadvertently or the false sac has eroded the posterior plate of the sternum. Once the sternum is opened and the pathology defined, the surgical procedures for repair are similar to those described in other sections.

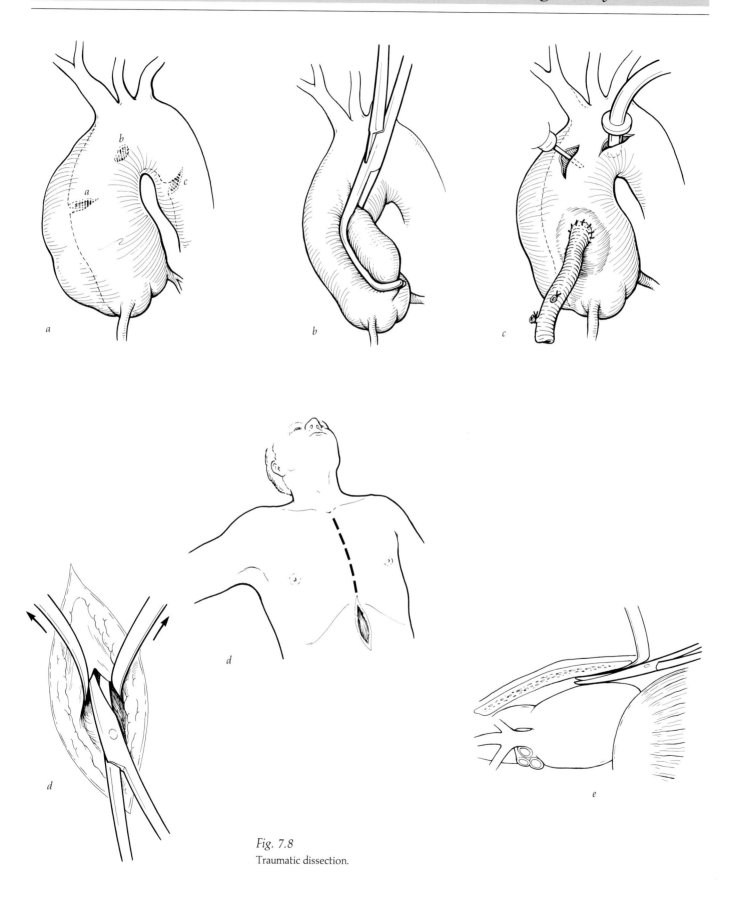

Fig. 7.8
Traumatic dissection.

Glue aortoplasty

Localized dissections of the ascending thoracic aorta such as those which follow cannulation or damage to the aorta during clamping or failure to incorporate the deeper layer of the aortic wall during saphenous vein bypass grafting (Fig. 7.9a) can be treated effectively with the glue aortoplasty technique described by Carpentier (1991a) using GRF glue.

The procedure can be performed with normal bypass technique if the lesion is readily accessible, such as in the proximal aorta. However, if the dissection occurs at the site of aortic cannulation or involves the aortic arch, femoral arterial cannulation and deep hypothermic circulatory arrest are necessary to obtain satisfactory exposure.

In the case of a dissection around a proximal anastomosis between a saphenous vein graft and the aorta, the saphenous vein is detached from the aortic wall and the diagnosis confirmed. A separate incision is made in the aorta to expose the dissection more widely (Fig. 7.9b). GRF glue is placed in the dissection sac and is kept dry by the placement of a distal clamp. The lumen of the aorta is then packed with a gauze swab or a large Foley catheter to compress the two layers for approximately 15 minutes. When the glue has hardened, the gauze swab is removed and the aortotomy for the saphenous vein is refashioned. The saphenous vein is reattached to the aorta and the aortotomy site is closed (Fig. 7.9c).

Special difficulties

GRF glue is very effective if it is confined rather than being allowed to spread down a long length of aorta. The technique, therefore, is best suited to localized dissections; however, more extensive dissection can be repaired using multiple clamps. Bleeding into the dissection site will wash out the glue and prevent hardening, resulting in failure to appose the dissection layers. For a more extensive dissection, formal resection and graft replacement may prove more satisfactory.

Aortic dissection with involvement of the aortic arch

Minor involvement of the aortic arch
Resection or anastomosis to the proximal aortic arch is a relatively simple extension of the previous technique described for tube graft repair of the dissection of the ascending thoracic aorta (Fig. 7.2a–g). Placement

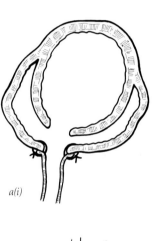

a(i)

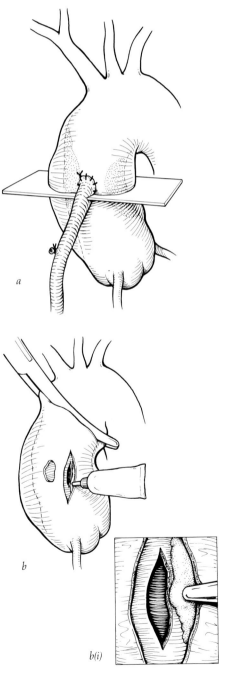

a

b

b(i)

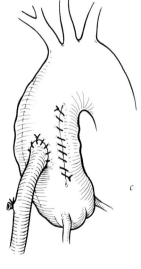

c

Fig. 7.9
Glue aortoplasty.

of the upper anastomosis in the proximal aortic arch may facilitate the aortic repair if the distal ascending thoracic aorta is involved. More extensive arch replacement is only necessary if there is major disruption of the aortic arch, branch occlusion or when the intimal tear commences in the arch itself.

Aortic dissection with extensive involvement of the aortic arch

Resection of the aortic arch for aortic dissection is required occasionally. Because of the technical difficulties and the risks of cerebral and other organ damage, the use of this procedure is usually limited to those patients who are younger, and have extensive dissections or a complication of an arch dissection. A primary tear in the arch, leakage or rupture from the aortic arch constitutes an indication for arch replacement. Gross disruption of the intimal flaps that obstruct the arch vessels can only be repaired by opening the aortic arch.

This procedure is performed under deep hypothermic circulatory arrest with retrograde cerebral perfusion and retrograde vital organ perfusion if it is anticipated that the procedure will be prolonged. Cannulation is via the right common femoral artery and femoral vein. Additional cannulae are placed in the left ventricle, coronary sinus and superior vena cava for the retrograde cerebral perfusion. Systemic cooling is continued until the temperature has been lowered to the required level. Cardiopulmonary bypass is discontinued and retrograde superior vena cava perfusion and inferior vena cava perfusion are commenced (see Ch. 5, p. 47).

The aortic arch is opened longitudinally along the anterior and left side. The incision is carried to the level of the subclavian artery: A transverse incision at either end increases the exposure to the aorta.

The distal aorta is repaired using a teflon sandwich or GRF glue (Fig. 7.10a). A graft of the appropriate size is chosen and sutured end to end to the repaired aorta (Fig. 6.5c). The graft

is then placed under tension and an oval segment of dacron removed from the superior surface of the graft corresponding to the innominate, left common carotid and left subclavian orifices (Fig. 7.10b). The side of the dacron graft is then anastomosed to the common orifice of the arch vessels commencing posteriorly and to the left of the subclavian artery and being completed anteriorly (Fig. 6.5f).

Retrograde cerebral perfusion is continued throughout. When the distal anastomoses are complete, the cardiopulmonary bypass is recommenced slowly to remove any embolic material from the lower circulation while the retrograde cerebral perfusion displaces air from the arch vessels. The aortic graft is then clamped and the cerebral perfusion discontinued. The patient is then rewarmed on full cardiopulmonary bypass. The proximal end of the dissection is repaired and the aortic root reconstructed with a valve conduit and coronary implantation (Fig. 6.5l) or with a simple graft (Fig. 7.10c) in a supracoronary position.

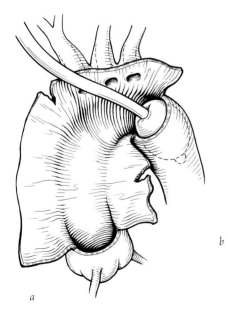

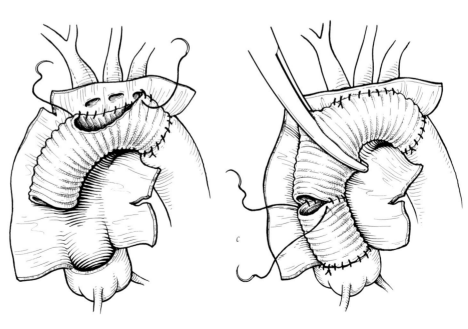

Fig. 7.10
Repair of aortic arch dissection.

The two grafts are measured and divided for the final anastomosis (Figs 6.5l and 7.10c). Prior to completion of this anastomosis, the left ventricular vent is discontinued, the heart filled with blood and any air evacuated through the graft suture line prior to closure. A vent is then placed in the dacron graft and the aortic cross-clamp released. Once haemostasis has been secured, the remaining dissection sac is loosely wrapped over the dacron graft.

TYPE B DISSECTIONS

Repair of descending thoracic aortic dissection with tube graft

Repair of a dissection of the descending thoracic aorta is usually performed electively rather than as an emergency, unlike dissections of the ascending thoracic aorta. Type B dissections (Fig. 7.11a) tend to occur in an older age group and are often associated with hypertension, kidney and lung disease. For that reason, the initial management is often conservative and surgery is performed when there is continuing chest pain, progressive dilatation of the false sac or leakage or rupture into the pleural space. Branch occlusion may also constitute an indication for surgical correction. The anatomy should be defined prior to reconstruction to determine which branches are filled from the true lumen and which are filled from the false lumen.

Control of the dissection process is achieved by placing in the upper thoracic aorta, a short segment interposition graft, which should include the intimal tear. The procedure is normally performed under left heart bypass or partial cardioplumonary bypass using femorofemoral cannulation. Some surgeons prefer to correct the lesion without bypass using a simple cross-clamp technique.

The surgical exposure is through a posterolateral thoracotomy in the fourth interspace. Extra exposure can be obtained at the upper end by dividing the costotransverse ligaments or the neck of the fifth rib. Care is taken in mobilizing the vagus nerve and the recurrent laryngeal branch from the aorta. The aorta is clamped above the entry site. Clamping the distal aortic arch between the left common carotid and left subclavian arteries will greatly increase the access to the upper descending thoracic aorta (Fig. 6.11d). A further clamp is placed in the mid-descending thoracic aortic level distally. The aneurysm sac is opened longitudinally and transected at either end (Fig. 7.11b). The false sac and true lumen are opened to display the intercostal arteries, which are oversewn from within. The two ends of the aorta are then repaired with either teflon or GRF glue (Fig. 7.11c). The lumen is packed with gauze or distended with a large Foley catheter to compress the dissected layers while the glue hardens (Fig. 7.11d). A graft is sutured to the upper end of the transected aorta using a continuous suture. The suture is usually commenced superiorly and to the left and the posterior wall sutured from within. The anastomosis is completed on the anterior wall (Fig. 7.11e).

The inferior anastomosis is then performed, with the posterior wall being completed prior to the anterior wall (Fig. 7.11e). (If one or more major branches fills from the false sac, a fenestration is performed in the distal suture line—see p. 78.) Prior to closure of the distal anastomosis, the aorta is flushed to remove any embolic material. A needle is then placed in the dacron graft and the distal clamp removed and any remaining air evacuated. Atriofemoral bypass is discontinued and when the distal aortic pressure is lower than the proximal pressure the proximal aortic clamp is released so that flow is directed distally. If the distal pressure is higher than the proximal pressure, it is possible that any remaining particulate matter could be directed into the cerebral circulation. Once the haemostasis has been completed, the remaining dissection sac is wrapped over the dacron graft.

If the proximal and distal aortic tissues are particularly friable, additional support can be given to the aorta adjacent to the suture lines by placing an 8 mm dacron vascular prosthesis secured with three or four interrupted sutures (Fig. 7.11f).

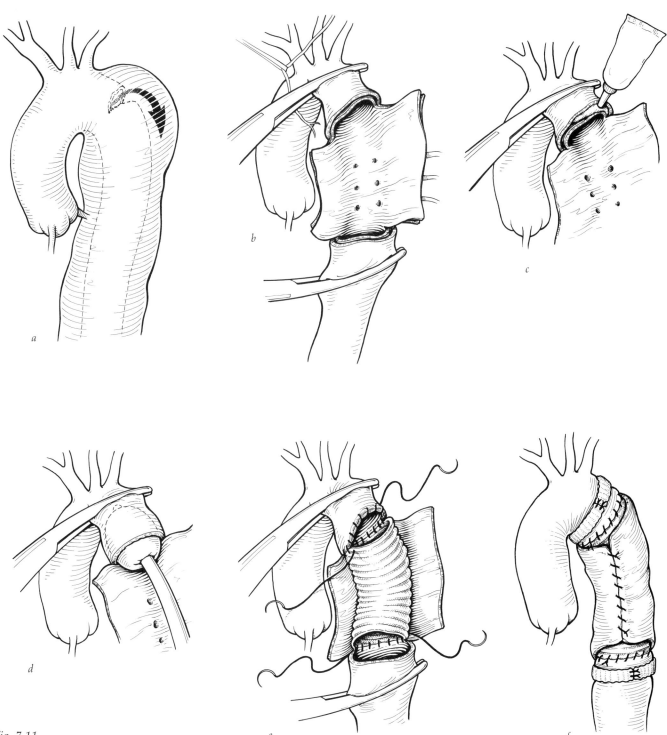

Fig. 7.11
Repair of descending thoracic aortic dissection.

Intraluminal grafting of an aortic dissection

The intraluminal graft was thought to be a major advance in the treatment of aortic dissection (Berger et al 1983, Serra et al 1989), because it could be implanted quickly and safely using a sutureless technique. Its use in the infrarenal aortic aneurysms is described on page 137. However, the intraluminal graft requires careful manipulation to be positioned correctly into the true lumen of the aorta. This technique requires mobilization of 2–3 cm of aorta above and below the site of transection to allow appropriate implantation. The graft itself is bulky and often results in the lumen of the graft being smaller than the lumen of the aorta. The late angiographic findings sometimes reveal a residual leak around the nylon ties, further complicating its use.

Surgical technique
Intraluminal grafting of the descending thoracic aorta can be performed without bypass or using a simple cross-clamping technique. Left heart bypass or a femorofemoral bypass technique may afford more stable perfusion of the distal circulation during insertion.

The aorta is opened longitudinally and the descending thoracic aorta is clamped above and below the site of entry. The aorta is opened to expose the intimal tear. A valve sizer is introduced into the true lumen to measure the diameter. It is important not to use a prosthesis which is too wide as this will cause difficulty during insertion.

Insertion and placement of the graft are aided by three or four traction sutures placed through the lip of the intraluminal graft and then back into the true lumen of the aorta and then through the aortic wall (Fig. 7.12a). The graft is advanced through the true lumen and the stay sutures tied over small pledgets. A similar procedure is performed with the distal end. Nylon tapes 6 mm wide are placed around the aorta at the level of the groove in the upper and lower ends of the intraluminal prosthesis and tied securely (Fig. 7.12b).

The use of the intraluminal graft is restricted to areas where sufficient aorta is available, such as in the mid-ascending thoracic aorta or in the mid-descending thoracic aorta. If difficulty is obtained introducing the rigid end of the intraluminal graft, the ring can be removed and the graft can be anastomosed directly to the aorta.

Thromboexclusion

The principle of the thromboexclusion technique described by Carpentier is to implant a 20 mm dacron graft between two non-dissected areas (Carpentier et al 1981, Carpentier 1991b). A permanent aortic cross-clamp is placed on the descending aorta just distal to the left subclavian artery so that the flows goes from the ascending thoracic aorta through the graft, into the abdominal aorta and retrogradely to the thoracic aorta. The false lumen is thus compressed, allowing it to thrombose gradually so that collaterals have time to develop.

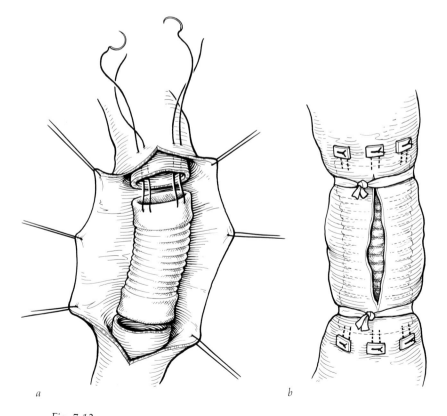

a   *b*

Fig. 7.12
Intraluminal grafting.

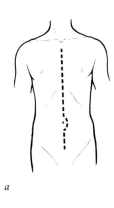

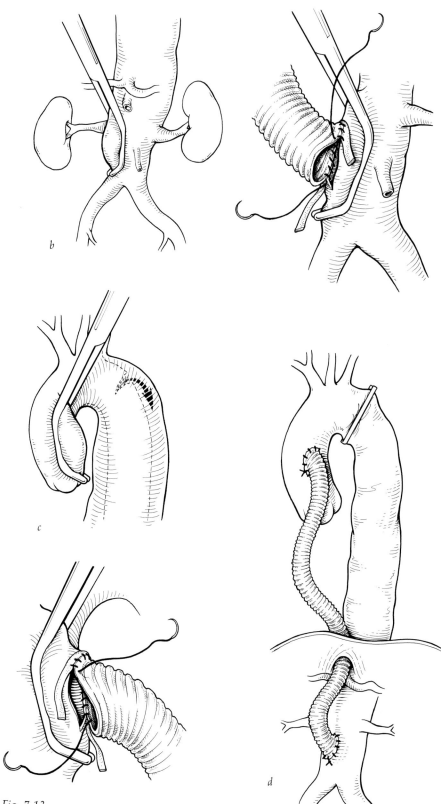

The technique is performed without the use of cardiopulmonary bypass and the need for an extracorporeal shunt. The approach is via median sternotomy, which is continued to the lower abdomen (Fig. 7.13a).

A 20 mm gelatin-impregnated dacron graft is anastomosed end to side into a non-diseased portion of the abdominal aorta, which is cross-clamped under heparinization. The edges of the aortotomy are reinforced with a teflon strip and the anastomosis is performed with a continuous suture (Fig. 7.13b). The graft is passed superiorly behind the stomach, through the diaphragm anterior to the vena cava and positioned within the right pleural cavity lateral to the heart. The graft is then passed through the pericardium to the level of the ascending thoracic aorta and anastomosed to the ascending thoracic aorta using a partial occlusion clamp, again using teflon strips (Fig. 7.13c).

A permanent clamp or row of staples is placed across the aorta distal to the left subclavian artery (Fig. 7.13d). This is facilitated by the use of temporary cross-clamping of the aorta distal to the left subclavian artery. Adequate pulsation of the abdominal arteries is carefully checked before the sternum and abdomen are closed.

Fig. 7.13
Thromboexclusion for type B dissection. (Redrawn from Carpentier 1991b).

REFERENCES

Berger R L, Romero L, Chaudhry A G, Dobnik D B 1983 Graft replacement of the thoracic aorta with sutureless technique. Annals of Thoracic Surgery 35: 231–239

Cabrol C, Pavie A, Gandjbakhch I et al 1981 Complete replacement of the ascending aorta with reimplantation of the coronary arteries. Journal of Thoracic and Cardiovascular Surgery 81: 309–315

Cabrol C, Pavie A, Mesnildrey P et al 1986 Long-term results with total replacement of the ascending aorta and reimplantation of the coronary arteries. Journal of Thoracic and Cardiovascular Surgery 91: 17–25

Carpentier A 1991a 'Glue aortoplasty' as an alternative to resection and grafting for the treatment of aortic dissection. Seminars in Thoracic and Cardiovascular Surgery 3: 213–214

Carpentier A 1991b Thromboexclusion: an alternative for type B dissection. Seminars in Thoracic and Cardiovascular Surgery (Floyd Loop) 3: 242–244

Carpentier A, Deloche A, Fabiani J N et al 1981 New surgical approach to aortic dissection: flow reversal and thromboexclusion. Journal of Thoracic and Cardiovascular Surgery 81: 659–668

Cooley D 1991 Experience with hypothermic circulatory arrest and the treatment of aneurysms of the ascending aortic arch. Seminars in Thoracic and Cardiovascular Surgery 3: 166–170

Crawford E S, Crawford J L, Stowe C I, Carey L, Hazim J S 1984 Total aortic replacement for chronic aortic dissection occurring in patients with and without Marfan's syndrome. Annals of Surgery 199: 358–362

Daily P O, Trueblood H W, Stinson E B, Wuerflein R D, Shumway N E 1970 Management of acute aortic dissections. Annals of Thoracic Surgery 10: 237–247

Erbel R, Engbergbing R, Daniel W, Roelandt J, Visser C, Rennollett H 1989 Echocardiography in the diagnosis of aortic dissection. Lancet i: 457–461

Hashimoto S, Kumada T, Osakada G et al 1989 Assessment of transesophageal Doppler echocardiography in dissecting aneurysm. Journal of the American College of Cardiology 14: 1253–1262

Hirst A E, Johns V J Jr, Kiame S W Jr 1958 Dissecting aneurysm of the aorta: review of 505 cases. Medicine (Baltimore) 37: 217–279

Livesay J J, Cooley D A, Duncan J M, Ott D A, Walker W E, Reul G J 1982 Open aortic anastomosis: improved results in the treatment of aneurysms of the aortic arch. Circulation (Suppl I) 66: 122–127

Miller D C 1991 Surgical management of acute aortic dissection. New data. Seminars in Thoracic and Cardiovascular Surgery 3: 225–237

Serra A J, McNicholas K W, Spagna P M, Karmilowicz N P, Lemole G M 1989 Replacement of the descending thoracic aorta with intraluminal ring graft. Annals of Thoracic Surgery 48: 689–692

Chapter 8

Thoracoabdominal aneurysm

Introduction

These patients present major challenges. This is not so much because of the technical problems in replacing a large segment of the aorta but more because of the difficulties of maintaining cardiac, renal and spinal cord function. The two critical times are the cross-clamping of the aorta, when it will be necessary to give vasodilator drugs to reduce the afterload on the left ventricle, and the time of declamping as severe hypotension may develop when the flow is restored to the visceral vessels. The postoperative period, too, requires expert intensive care to maintain homeostasis and prevent the development of complications.

CLASSIFICATION

The common feature of these aneurysms is involvement of the abdominal visceral branches. They have been classified by Crawford (1990) into four groups depending on the degree of involvement of the thoracic and abdominal aorta (Fig. 8.1).

An important key to these procedures is the understanding that the orifices of the four major visceral arteries (coeliac, superior mesenteric and both renal arteries) are close together and therefore are commonly dealt with in an identical manner. In the discussion which follows, the term 'visceral arteries' includes these four arteries.

INDICATIONS FOR OPERATION

Symptomatic patients should be offered operation if it is felt that their general condition permits. Asymptomatic patients should be offered surgery if they are otherwise in good health and if the aneurysm is greater than 5 cm diameter. The limited data on the natural history of these aneurysms suggest that rupture is common and occurred in half the patients who were treated non-operatively (Crawford & DeNatale 1986).

INVESTIGATIONS

Computed tomographic (CT) scanning should be performed to demonstrate the extent of the aneurysm. In many cases this must be carried out from the root of the aorta to the iliac arteries. Angiography is essential to demonstrate the origins of the visceral vessels.

The function of the heart, lungs and kidneys is carefully evaluated and corrected if necessary as outlined on page 11.

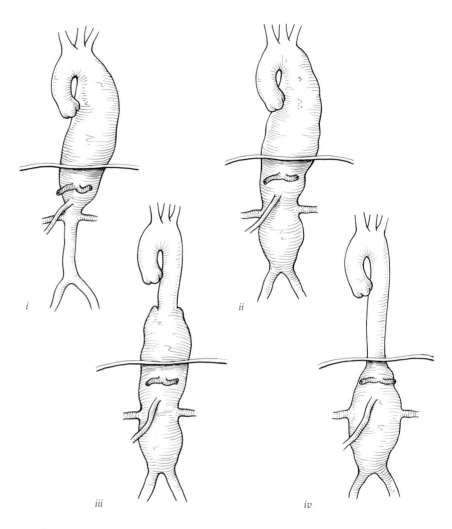

i   *ii*

iii   *iv*

Fig. 8.1
Types of thoracoabdominal aneurysms (after Crawford 1990).

Table 8.1

	Involvement of thoracic aorta	Involvement of abdominal aorta
Group i	More than half the descending thoracic aorta[a]	Proximal part, including visceral branches
Group ii	As in group i[a]	Visceral branches and distal abdominal aorta
Group iii	Less than half descending thoracic aorta	As in group ii
Group iv	Minimal involvement	As in groups ii and iii

[a] There is involvement of the ascending aorta ± the arch in 50% of these patients.

OPERATION

Preparation and monitoring

The account in this section is modified from that given by Crawford (1990). The most intensive monitoring is required for these patients. The details have been described on page 18 and include intravenous lines, urinary catheter, ECG and direct arterial pressure. A Swan–Ganz catheter will be inserted to enable the measurement of central venous pressure, pulmonary artery pressure, pulmonary capillary wedge pressure and cardiac output. Arterial blood gases will be measured as necessary.

A double-lumen endotracheal tube will be inserted to allow deflation of the left lung.

Details of the techniques for blood replacement are given on page 20. Crawford (1990) recommends the use of techniques allowing rapid autotransfusion, the liberal use of fresh frozen plasma and platelet transfusions before the development of coagulopathy. Fibrinolytic disturbances are corrected by infusing 6–40 units cryoprecipitate.

Mannitol 25 g is administered before application of the aortic clamp to produce an osmotic diuresis. To prevent acidosis following declamping, NaHCO$_3$ 0.05 meq/kg per minute is given during the period of aortic clamping.

Cardiopulmonary bypass, hypothermia (see Ch. 5) and anticoagulation with heparin may be used if the arch and thoracoabdominal segments are to be replaced at the same operation, in patients with very large aneurysms, if the proximal exposure is difficult or in case of injury to the aorta or pulmonary artery.

Incision

The patient is placed on the right side, with the left side elevated to make an angle of about 45° with the operating table. The left arm is supported on a stand (Fig. 8.2).

If the proximal aorta is involved the incision is made in the sixth intercostal space. In other cases the incision is made in the eighth intercostal space. After the costal margin has been divided, the abdominal incision is carried out extraperitoneally as far distally as necessary to control the arteries below the aneurysm. Details of this part of the incision are given on page 110.

Posteriorly, there is a choice to be made between staying anterior to the kidney and keeping the ureter laterally while continuing to mobilize the peritoneum medially or, more commonly, the kidney and ureter are carried forward with the peritoneum (Fig. 8.3). Using the latter approach allows the possibility of anastomosing the four visceral arteries as one patch.

The diaphragm is divided either radially or peripherally to the aortic hiatus. Division of the left crus exposes the aorta.

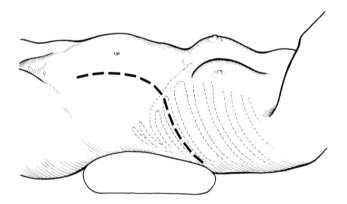

Fig. 8.2
Incision.

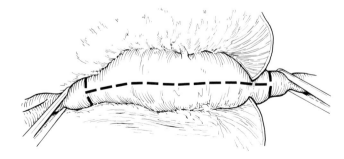

Fig. 8.3
View from left side after mobilization of abdominal viscera. The divided left crus and left leaf of the diaphragm are shown.

Proximal anastomosis

The left lung is collapsed. The area chosen for the proximal anastomosis will be just above the aneurysm. The pleura over the aorta is divided and the aorta gently dissected from the surrounding structures and encircled with a tape placed in the jaws of a clamp. Depending on the level of the dissection, the structures to be avoided include the pulmonary artery, the left recurrect laryngeal nerve and the oesophagus. Dissection close to the wall of the aorta will minimize the chances of injury to adjacent structures. Careful dissection posteriorly is necessary to avoid damage to the intercostal arteries.

A clamp is placed across the proximal aorta and closed gradually while the anaesthetist monitors cardiac function and blood pressure and administers vasodilators (glyceryl trinitrate or sodium nitroprusside) to avoid proximal hypertension.

When the aorta has been clamped proximally, the distal iliac or aortic clamp(s) are applied. The proximal part of the wall of the aneurysm is opened, thrombus is removed and the proximal aorta prepared for anastomosis. The aneurysm is opened sufficiently to display the area of the anastomosis and any intercostal arteries in the vicinity. Back-bleeding from the visceral, lumbar and intercostal arteries is controlled by packing. A graft with zero porosity is inserted. A woven Dacron graft has been most commonly used but the modern, impregnated, knitted grafts are now preferred. The proximal end of the graft is sutured to the aorta using the technique described in Figures 10.9–10.13.

Intercostal/lumbar vessels

Paraplegia is a catastrophic complication of surgery on the thoracoabdominal aorta. The possible mechanisms have been described on page 50. The best strategy to avoid it seems to be to incorporate into the graft vessels arising in the area of the proximal anastomosis. As a general rule, all significant intercostal and lumbar vessels should be reattached. Two techniques are illustrated. Figure 8.4 shows the modification of the anastomosis to incorporate two pairs of lumbar arteries. If necessary the arteries may be controlled temporarily by inserting small balloon catheters. An extension of this approach to include four pairs of arteries is shown in Figure 8.5.

Alternatively the arteries may be reimplanted into a separate defect cut into the graft (Fig. 8.6). After completion and testing of the proximal anastomosis, tension is applied to the graft and a hole cut into it to correspond to the area of aortic wall containing the orifices of the intercostal vessels to be incorporated. The graft must be pulled tight to mimic the extension of the graft which occurs when blood flow is restored. The proximal clamp (not shown) may at this stage be placed distal to the anastomosis. It is safer to cut only the proximal half to two-thirds of the defect at this stage. Suturing starts at the proximal end or a convenient place in the proximal half of the posterior wall. The posterior wall is sutured from within the aneurysm. The suture line is finished after removal of any occluding balloon catheters and flushing the graft. The proximal clamp is removed from the aorta and placed on the graft below the suture line just completed.

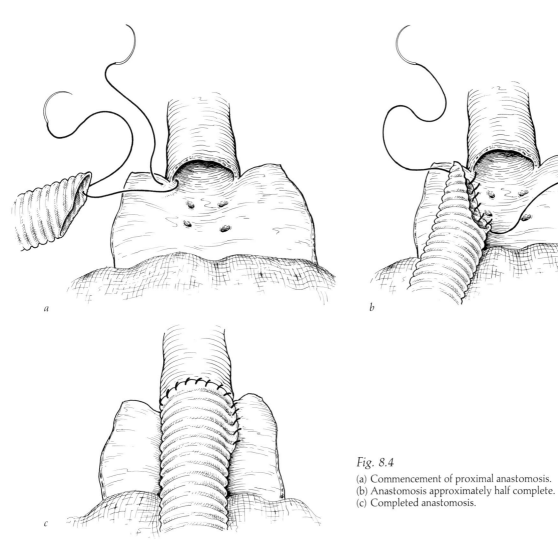

a

b

c

Fig. 8.4

(a) Commencement of proximal anastomosis.
(b) Anastomosis approximately half complete.
(c) Completed anastomosis.

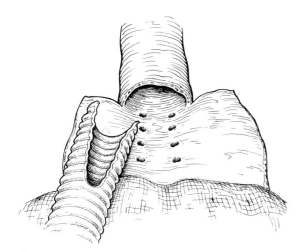

Fig. 8.5

Incorporation of intercostal arteries in anastomosis.

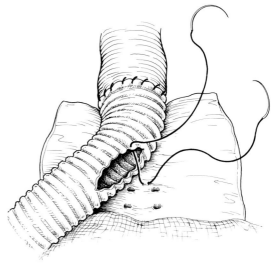

Fig. 8.6

Reimplantation of distal intercostal arteries.

Visceral arteries

The incision is extended along the length of the aneurysm. Thrombus in the lumen is removed and the orifices of the visceral arteries come into view. Lumbar arteries may be oversewn. The orifices of the visceral vessels are occluded with balloon catheters if there is significant back-bleeding. The technique of anastomosis is similar to that used for the reimplantation of the intercostal vessels. The coeliac, superior mesenteric and right renal arteries can be reimplanted as one patch. Figure 8.7 shows the relative position of the orifices which lie in the anterior wall of the aneurysm. The suture line is begun at the proximal end with a large bite through the wall of the aorta. After tying the first stitch, the graft is rolled posteriorly and the posterior wall of the anastomosis is being sutured from within the lumen (Fig. 8.8). Figure 8.9 shows the anastomosis almost complete.

If the incision in the aorta has been made in front of the left renal artery, this vessel will need to be reimplanted into a separate defect cut into the graft (Fig. 8.10). A clamp is placed so that blood flow can be restored to the remaining visceral arteries while this is carried out.

Distal anastomosis

This is carried out end to end as described on page 129. It is not usually necessary to insert a bifurcated graft but the techniques described on page 134 may be used as necessary. If the infrarenal abdominal aorta is not dilated (type I aneurysm), the distal anastomosis may be fashioned to include the visceral arteries (Fig. 8.11).

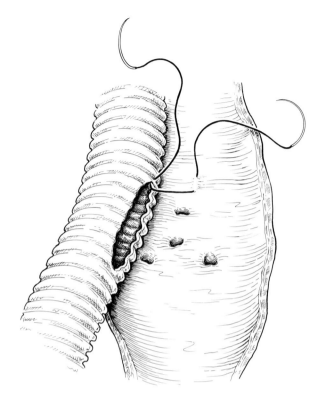

Fig. 8.7
Commencement of anastomosis of visceral vessels.

REFERENCES

Crawford E S 1990 Thoraco-abdominal and proximal aortic replacement for extensive aortic aneurysmal disease. In: Greenhalgh R M, Mannick J A, Powell J T (eds) The cause and management of aneurysms. W B Saunders, London, pp 351–372

Crawford E S, DeNatale R W 1986 Thoracoabdominal aortic aneurysm: observations regarding the natural course of the disease. Journal of Vascular Surgery 3: 578–582

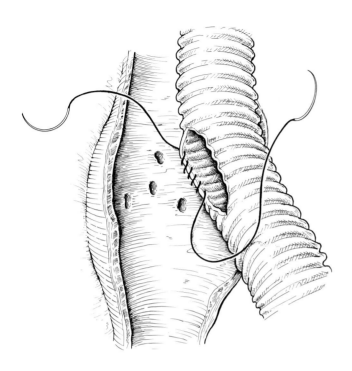

Fig. 8.8
Suturing posterior wall of anastomosis.

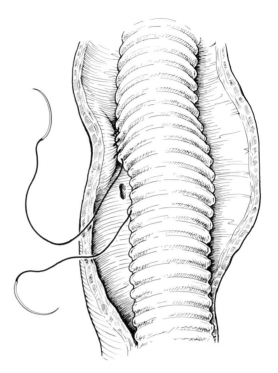

Fig. 8.9
Anastomosis almost complete.

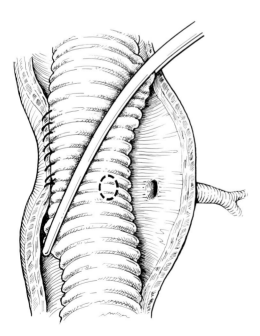

Fig. 8.10
The graft is clamped and blood flow restored to the three implanted visceral arteries. The site for implantation of the left renal artery is shown.

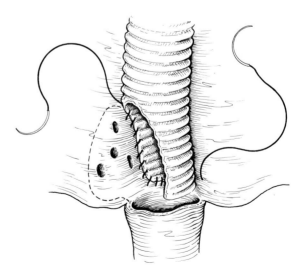

Fig. 8.11
Lower anastomosis fashioned to include visceral arteries.

Chapter 9

Retroperitoneal approach

Introduction

A variety of retroperitoneal approaches may be used to gain access to aneurysm of the aorta or its major branches. These include:

1. Thoracoabdominal aneurysm (see previous section)
2. Abdominal aortic aneurysm

a. Involving visceral branches
b. Not involving visceral branches
3. Iliac aneurysm (see p. 197).

The retroperitoneal approach was used for the first replacement of the abdominal aorta by Dubost in 1951 and, by 1963, Rob was able to report its use in 500 patients with aortic or iliac disease. It was anticipated that avoiding intraperitoneal dissection would reduce the incidence of respiratory and intestinal complications, but this was not verified in the only prospective randomized trial comparing the two approaches that has been reported to date (Cambria et al 1990).

INDICATIONS

This approach should be considered in the following conditions:

1. The 'hostile' abdomen, where there have been multiple previous intra-abdominal procedures, in the presence of intra-abdominal sepsis or intestinal or urinary stoma.
2. Previous aortic operations.
3. Juxtarenal or suprarenal aneurysms.
4. Visceral artery disease, especially coexisting left renal artery stenosis.
5. Obesity.
6. Inflammatory abdominal aortic aneurysm.

PREOPERATIVE ASSESSMENT

This should include:

1. Aortography with particular attention to the right renal and right iliac arteries. Abnormalities of the right renal vessels may contraindicate the retroperitoneal approach to the aorta because of difficulty in dissecting and exposing these arteries. If access to the right common iliac artery is needed, a second incision in the right iliac fossa may be made.
2. Computed tomographic scan should be performed to exclude the presence of a right iliac aneurysm.

OPERATION

Position of patient

For exposure of the aorta, the patient may be placed in one of two alternative positions:

1. The upper part of the trunk is rotated approximately 45° toward the right side while the lower trunk and limbs remain supine (Fig. 8.2). A small sandbag may be placed above the right iliac crest to separate the lower rib cage from the iliac crest (Anderson et al 1990).

2. The patient is placed on the right side with the chest fixed in the true lateral position but the lower half of the body is allowed to rotate to the left so that the trunk is twisted (Williams et al 1980). A sandbag is necessary to support the left buttock.

In either position the space between iliac crest and ribs may be opened up by breaking the operating table. Rotation of the table towards or away from the surgeon allows access to either the groin or the retroperitoneal aorta.

Incision

A number of incisions have been described:

1. From midway between umbilicus and pubic symphysis and extended in a curvilinear manner 5 cm superior to the anterior superior iliac spine posteriorly to the 12th rib or into the 11th intercostal space.
2. From the lateral border of the rectus muscle about 5 cm below the umbilicus to the 10th or 11th interspace in the posterior axillary line. (The rib may or may not be removed.) The incision may be extended inferiorly as far as the pubis.

Less commonly, a midline or a transverse left upper abdominal incision may be used.

With all incisions the muscles are divided in the line of the incision to expose the peritoneum (Fig. 9.1). The fingers are shown inserted through an incision in the internal oblique and transversus abdominus muscles. This is best performed close to the costal margin where the distance between the muscles and the peritoneum is greatest. Division of the muscles is completed while the fingers protect the underlying peritoneum. The retroperitoneal space is entered laterally and the peritoneum is swept off the abdominal wall in a medial direction. Anteriorly the dissection

proceeds to the lateral border of the rectus sheath. Medially the peritoneum is thinner and more densely attached to the overlying fascia. Small holes in the peritoneum are repaired with absorbable sutures. The dissection may be carried out either in front of or behind the kidney (Fig. 9.2).

In operations on the infrarenal aorta the major structure limiting access to the lateral aspect of the whole of the infrarenal aorta is a vein which joins the left renal vein to the lumbar or azygous systems (Fig. 9.3). This vein needs to be ligated and divided to allow the left kidney to be pushed forward and so optimize exposure of the juxtarenal aorta. The position of the left ureter and left renal artery is shown. It is more difficult to completely encircle the aorta with the retroperitoneal approach and so rather than risk damage to the vena cava and lumbar vessels by blind passage of a clamp it is best to place a straight clamp across the aorta after exposing it anteriorly and posteriorly as shown in the figure.

Mobilization of the peritoneum over the distal aorta and right common iliac artery is helped by dividing the inferior mesenteric artery. Control of the left common iliac artery by conventional methods is straightforward but because of the limited exposure of the right common iliac artery intraoperative control of back-bleeding may be obtained best with a Foley catheter (Fig. 9.4).

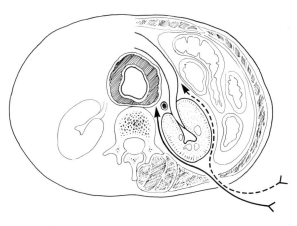

Fig. 9.2
Transverse section to show plane of dissection.

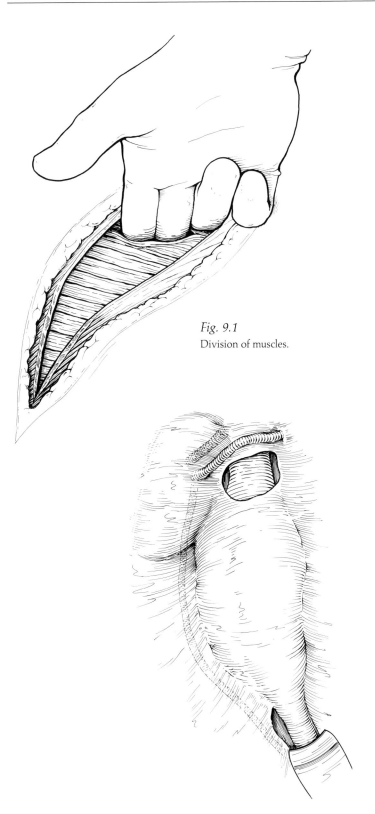

Fig. 9.1
Division of muscles.

Fig. 9.3
View of field with kidney retracted. Window of aorta exposed over neck of aneurysm.

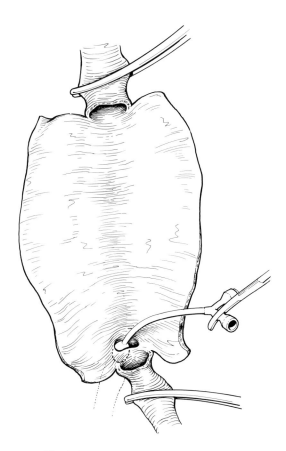

Fig. 9.4
View inside aneurysm. Foley catheter in orifice of right common iliac artery.

The retroperitoneal approach gives excellent exposure of the left iliac arteries but limited exposure of the right iliac artery, and makes tunnelling of an aortobifemoral graft more difficult. In occlusive disease it is usually possible to sweep the peritoneum off the right common iliac artery and to complete the tunnel to the femoral artery by creating a track on the anterior aspect of the external iliac artery. This is possible by using a bimanual technique from the groin and abdominal incision, taking care that both index fingers remain close to the external iliac artery, thus ensuring that the ureter and bowel are not damaged.

When the patient has a right iliac aneurysm and a bi-iliac graft is planned it is usually necessary to make a separate incision in the right flank (Fig. 9.5) and an extraperitoneal exposure of the common iliac bifurcation (see section 198).

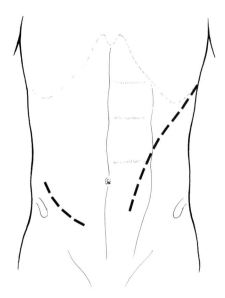

Fig. 9.5
Separate incision in right iliac fossa.

After administration of heparin, clamps are applied and the aneurysm opened. The operation then proceeds in the standard manner. At the end of the procedure the wall of the aneurysm may be sutured over the graft. This is not essential because, in contrast to the transperitoneal approach, the duodenum and small bowel are a safe distance away from the graft.

If there is concern about the viability of the intestine, it is a simple matter to open the peritoneum and inspect the bowel at any stage of the operation.

The right renal artery is inaccessible beyond its orifice and so only orifice lesions associated with a poststenotic dilatation are suitable for endarterectomy by this approach.

OTHER APPLICATIONS

Juxtarenal and suprarenal aneurysms
The higher the extent of the aneurysm the higher the interspace that the incision is centred over, so that for aneurysms extending to the level of the coeliac axis an incision through the eighth interspace will be adequate and for aneurysms involving the descending thoracic aorta an incision through the sixth interspace is recommended (see page 101). It is not necessary to excise the rib, but exposure is improved by doing so. Once the pleural cavity has been entered, the diaphragm is divided. It has been the conventional teaching that peripheral division of the diaphragm, 1 cm from its attachment to the ribs, results in less denervation than radial incision. However, some experienced surgeons are unable to demonstrate any difference in outcome between the two approaches.

The key to the exposure of the aorta above the renal artery is the division of the left crus of the diaphragm (Fig. 9.6). This arises from the anterior aspect of the bodies of the upper two or three lumbar vertebrae and thus may extend down to or below the origin of the renal arteries. Control of the supracoeliac aorta may be obtained by dividing the crus in the line of its fibres and entering the plane around the aorta. At this level, there is thin areolar tissue and the aortic wall is soft. Thus it is relatively simple and quick to obtain sufficient exposure to place a clamp across the aorta.

Division of the distal part of the crus will display the origins of the coeliac and superior mesenteric arteries.

The technique for performance of anastomoses at this level is described in Chapter 13.

Ruptured abdominal aortic aneurysm
Some authors have considered this approach contraindicated in cases of ruptured abdominal aortic aneurysm, but others have advocated it as a method of gaining rapid control above the aneurysm (Chang et al 1988). When this approach is used for a case of rupture of the infrarenal aorta the first step is to insert the hand along the diaphragm to reach the crus and underlying supracoeliac aorta which is then compressed with one hand while the crus is divided to allow application of an aortic clamp. The infrarenal aorta is then exposed and another clamp applied above the neck of the aneurysm, allowing removal of the supracoeliac clamp.

Exposure of the origins of the coeliac and superior mesenteric arteries
The origin of the coeliac artery can be displayed by division of the left crus and the dense tissue containing nerves and lymphatics around the aorta. The proximal trunk of the superior mesenteric artery before branches arise can be isolated by this exposure although it will not be necessary to divide fibres of the diaphragm. A length of 5–10 cm can be obtained (Saifi et al

1990). When these vessels are to be exposed, access is better if the dissection takes place in the plane anterior to the kidney.

CLOSURE

The diaphragm, if divided, is sutured. The costal margin may be approximated with strong sutures. Alternatively, the adjacent margins of the divided costal margin may be resected to prevent them rubbing together. If the pleura has been opened, a tube is placed in the pleural space to promote rapid full inflation of the lung. A small hole in the pleura, made during an extrapleural approach, may be sutured without the need for intrapleural drainage.

Retractors are removed and the peritoneum allowed to fall back into the paravertebral gutter. The muscles should be repaired in two layers: a deep layer of interrupted sutures in the internal oblique and transversus abdominus muscles and a continuous layer to the aponeurosis of the external oblique muscle (Fig. 9.7).

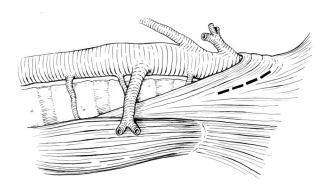

Fig. 9.6
Anatomy of left crus of the diaphragm showing site of incision for control of supracoeliac aorta.

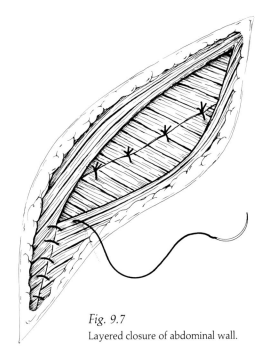

Fig. 9.7
Layered closure of abdominal wall.

REFERENCES

Anderson C B, Allen B T, Sicard G A 1990 The retroperitoneal approach to abdominal aneurysms. Surgery Annual 22: 281–298
Cambria R P, Brewster D C, Abbott W M et al 1990 Transperitoneal versus retroperitoneal approach for aortic reconstruction: a randomized prospective study. Journal of Vascular Surgery 11: 314–325
Chang B B, Paty P K, Shah D M, Leather R P 1988 Selective use of retroperitoneal exposure in the emergency treatment of ruptured and symptomatic abdominal aortic aneurysms. American Journal of Surgery 156: 108–110
Saifi J, Shah D M, Chang B B, Kaufman J L, Leather R P 1990 Left retroperitoneal exposure for distal mesenteric artery repair. Journal of Cardiovascular Surgery 31: 629–633
Williams G M, Ricotta J, Zinner M, Burdick J 1980 The extended retroperitoneal approach for treatment of extensive atherosclerosis of the aorta and renal vessels. Surgery 88: 846–855

ABDOMINAL AORTIC ANEURYSM

Chapter 10

Elective abdominal aortic aneurysm

Introduction

There is good evidence that the incidence of abdominal aortic aneurysm is increasing (Castleden et al 1985, Thomas & Stewart 1988). The use of screening studies has demonstrated that asymptomatic aneurysm may be present in 5.4% of males over the age 65–74 years (Collin et al 1988), 5% of patients with coronary artery disease (Thurmond 1986) and 10% of patients with peripheral atherosclerosis (Cabellon et al 1983). Screening of siblings of affected patients will probably result in more patients being referred for surgery (Webster et al 1991). In the USA ruptured abdominal aortic aneurysm ranks tenth as a cause of death for males older than 55 years.

The increased safety of aneurysm repair in recent years is only partly due to refinements in surgical technique. There have been major improvements in care at all stages of the process:

1.   Preoperative—assessment of cardiac function and screening for coronary artery disease (see p. 10).
2.   Intraoperative (see p. 18)—monitoring of cardiac function; autologous blood transfusion; pharmacological control of the circulation.
3.   Postoperative—respiratory support and monitoring in intensive care units.

CLINICAL FEATURES

The presentation of aortic aneurysm is classified under three headings:

1.   Asymptomatic—many patients are referred because the aneurysm has been felt on palpation of the abdomen during a routine examination. Increasingly, patients are referred following ultrasound or computed tomographic (CT) examination of the abdomen performed for some other reason.
2.   Symptomatic—the patient may complain of back pain which is indistinguishable from musculoskeletal pain. The history may extend for months or years. Sometimes the complaint is of central abdominal pain or the pulsating mass may be felt. The patient may present acutely with symptoms suggestive of rupture but without haemodynamic instability, although there may have been a period of hypotension at the onset of the pain.
3.   Ruptured—The classic triad of features of back pain, a pulsatile abdominal mass and hypotension. This syndrome is difficult to overlook. The second common pattern is of renal colic as the haematoma dissects through the retroperitoneal tissues on one side. Sometimes a mass is palpable in an iliac fossa. There are less acute presentations when the patient has been admitted to hospital for some time before the diagnosis becomes obvious with circulatory collapse (see p. 141).
4.   Rare presentations include aortocaval fistula (see p. 163), aortoenteric fistula (see p. 226) and atheroembolism—the 'blue toe syndrome'.

DIAGNOSTIC TESTS

Investigations are performed to determine the presence of an aneurysm and to provide data necessary to plan an operation (see p. 12).

Is there an aneurysm present?
In an outpatient setting this is best answered by ultrasound examination. This method has been used for screening populations and for following the rate of growth of unoperated aneurysms.

Does it involve the renal arteries?
In preparing for operation, this is the most important question which the surgeon wants answered. A CT scan may give the answer but tends to show that the aneurysm is higher than it really is. A report which indicates that the aneurysm is infrarenal can be relied on. A CT scan report which indicates that the aneurysm is close to the renal arteries usually means that it is safely infrarenal. If more information is required an arteriogram may be performed: using selective criteria this may only be necessary in 20% of cases (Todd et al 1991). This may be difficult to interpret because it only displays the lumen of the vessel; as a consequence, the extent of the aneurysm may be underestimated.

Has the aneurysm ruptured?
If the patient is haemodynamically unstable no further investigations should be performed. However, if the patient is stable, it is important to determine if the aneurysm has ruptured or not. CT scanning is the best way of determining this. For discussion of this issue see page 143.

Disease of the visceral and renal vessels which are not involved in the aneurysm is almost always incidental in the treatment of the aneurysm. However, if there is evidence of symptomatic vascular disease of the renal artery (manifest by hypertension or renal failure) or of the mesenteric circulation, preoperative angiography should be performed so that the visceral vascular lesions may be treated on their merits. Symptoms of peripheral ischaemia should be investigated by angiography.

INDICATIONS FOR OPERATION

Symptoms from the aneurysm are believed to herald rupture, although this may be delayed (e.g. for months). Symptomatic patients should be offered operation. Patients presenting with urgent symptoms should be investigated as outlined on page 143 and, if the aneurysm is shown to be intact, arrangements made for operation on the next available elective list.

Difficult decisions arise in patients who are asymptomatic. In general, operation is offered to patients who have an aneurysm which is 5.0 cm or more in diameter and who have a life expectancy of 2 years or more. Chronological age is not a barrier to operation (see p. 10). If the patient does not have ischaemic heart disease, rupture of the aneurysm is the commonest cause of death. In the presence of ischaemic heart disease, this is the major cause of death. In some patients the ischaemic heart disease is correctable with coronary artery bypass grafting. In many cases there are difficult decisions in balancing the risk of rupture, which is predominantly determined by the size of the aneurysm, against the risks of surgery, which are largely determined by the state of the coronary arteries and the general condition of the patient. For aneurysms between 4.5 and 5.0 cm, operation may be advised in any of the following circumstances:

1.   Age < 55 years.
2.   If the cardiac risk is low.
3.   If there is evidence of rapid expansion.
4.   If there is a family history of aortic aneurysm.
5.   If there have been complications of the aneurysm, e.g. embolism.
6.   If the patient lives in an area remote from the care which will be required should the aneurysm rupture.

PREOPERATIVE PREPARATION

The preoperative investigations are performed to determine the patient's general fitness for operation and the anatomy of the aneurysm. The high prevalence of coronary artery disease in these patients has led to the development of protocols to identify coronary artery disease which may jeopardize the safety of the operation. These issues are discussed on page 10.

PERIOPERATIVE CARE

The major aim of the perioperative care is to maintain the stability of the circulation as outlined on page 18.

Prophylactic antibiotics should be given as described on page 12.

OPERATION

Skin preparation and draping
Skin preparation involves the area from the nipples to the knees. It is necessary to allow access to the femoral arteries. The most superficial of the lower drapes is placed over the pubis in such a manner that it may be folded back to allow exposure of the femoral arteries if necessary. Some surgeons prepare the whole length of both legs and expose the feet, which are covered with transparent bags. The return of the circulation to the feet can be observed after the clamps are removed.

Incision
The most common incision is through the midline. This has the advantages of speed of access and being made in an avascular area. (The use of the retroperitoneal approach is described on p. 109.) The incision is made from the xiphoid process to near the pubis. In the upper part of the incision, the fatty tissue in the falciform ligament is encountered after incision of the linea alba. If this fatty tissue is swept to the right, the thin peritoneal membrane is encountered and this can be divided without the bleeding which occurs if the fatty tissue is divided directly. The maximum proximal exposure is obtained if the incision extends into the groove between the xiphoid process and the ribs. In this narrow space the xiphoid branch of the superior epigastric artery will usually need to be coagulated. The middle part of the incision skirts the umbilicus and continues distally, dividing in the midline the fascia between the bellies of the rectus abdominus muscle. At the lower end of the incision care must be taken not to damage the bladder.

An exploratory laparotomy is performed according to the surgeon's preferred routine. It is convenient to examine the supracolic compartment first while applying gentle traction to the greater omentum. The infracolic compartment is exposed by placing the omentum and transverse colon over the lower end of the sternum. The appendix and right colon are inspected and palpated and the small bowel is eviscerated over the right side of the wound, thus exposing the left colon and pelvis which are examined similarly.

Eviscerating the small bowel will expose the aneurysm. The small bowel may be kept away from the operative field in one of several ways. The bowel may be left in the abdomen and excluded by means of packs. This gives adequate exposure if there is a small aneurysm. More commonly the bowel is kept outside the abdomen and placed in a transparent, draw-string bag or covered with damp packs.

Retraction is maintained ideally with a fixed-frame retractor. Two blades retract the sides of the wound. A damp pack is placed over the transverse colon as far down as the root of the mesentery and a Deaver or similar retractor placed over it (Fig. 10.1). At this stage, the retractor should be held by an assistant.

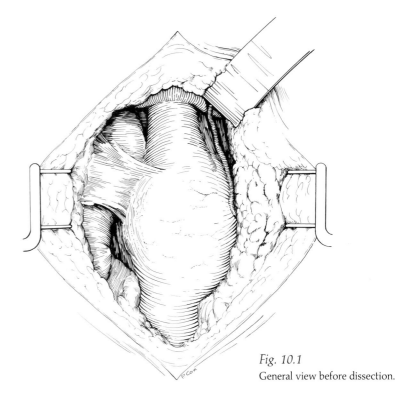

Fig. 10.1
General view before dissection.

Dissection of the aorta

The initial part of the operation involves controlling the arteries above and below the aneurysm. The first step is the mobilization of the duodenum from the aorta. Dissection begins at a convenient location to the left of the third part of the duodenum. The duodenum is lifted forwards and the peritoneum and loose areolar tissue behind it is divided. Superiorly, the vessels in the suspensory ligament of the duodenum (of Treitz) may need to be divided. Inferiorly, the dissection stops as the inferior vena cava is encountered to the right of the aorta. The duodenum is displaced to the right, covered with a damp pack and retracted with a broad-bladed retractor.

Next the area of the neck of the aneurysm is dissected. The upper limit of this dissection is the left renal vein. Dissection begins over the proximal part of the aneurysm (Fig. 10.2) and continues proximally in a plane as close to the aneurysm wall as possible. This fibro-fatty tissue which contains lymphatics and blood vessels becomes thicker as the renal vein is approached (Fig. 10.3). The dissection is aided by careful retraction of the root of the transverse mesocolon, which tends to lift the tissues forward and open up the space. In this area there may be large lymphatic channels which should be clipped or ligated. The blue renal vein should be encountered in the midline. Extra space for this dissection can be obtained by dividing the inferior mesenteric vein as it passes towards the root of the transverse mesocolon.

The degree to which it is necessary to dissect the renal veins varies. Figure 10.4 shows the anatomy of the branches of the left renal vein. In all cases the inferior border of the vein should be dissected as far as the inferior vena cava on the right, and to the left of the aorta. The gonadal vein and tributaries from the kidney to the left renal vein will be encountered. (For a detailed account of venous anomalies, see p. 172.) In an aneurysm which is close to the renal arteries, both surfaces of the renal vein should be dissected and the vein encircled with a sling. The gonadal vein should be divided between ligatures. The left adrenal vein entering the superior surface of the renal vein should also be ligated and divided. Additional mobility of the renal vein can be obtained by dissecting and dividing the tributary which runs back to the lumbar venous plexus. This dissection maximizes access to the aorta in the region of the renal arteries, because dissection can be carried out both above and below the renal vein.

The posterior dissection is facilitated by the aorta inclining forwards away from the vertebral column as it enters the aneurysm. This provides a 'window' of loose areolar tissue through which a clamp can be placed and is indicated by the asterisk in Figure 10.3. At the area of the junction of the renal vein and the inferior vena cava, a plane of loose areolar and fatty tissue begins to open up. This should be explored with the tip of an index finger. With gentle finger dissection the finger can pass at least to the midline behind the aorta. Firm strands binding the aorta to the vertebra can be felt. These are lumbar arteries and must not be disrupted because the bleeding produced is very difficult to control. It is usually possible for the tip of the index finger to feel a path between adjacent pairs of lumbar arteries. In some cases the finger will pass easily to the left of the aorta, in others an area can be identified through which a clamp can be passed.

A similar dissection is performed on the left side of the aorta, below the renal vein. Extra space can be obtained by dividing the fibro-fatty tissues on the left anterolateral aspect of the aorta. The inferior mesenteric vein may be ligated at this stage. At the end of this dissection it is often possible for index fingers passed from left and right, to meet behind the aorta. A large curved clamp (with jaws closed) is passed through the channel thus created and a tape inserted in its tip (Fig. 10.5). This tape is pulled through and the ends secured in an artery clip. This clamp should be passed from right to left in order to minimize the chances of damage to the inferior vena cava.

Not all surgeons insist on the passage of a tape behind the aorta. Avoiding this step removes the chance of damaging lumbar arteries and veins behind the aorta where access is very difficult. The occluding clamp is placed vertically and the aorta is occluded from side to side. In this method, the area in the midline posteriorly may be more difficult to suture accurately than when a transverse clamp is used.

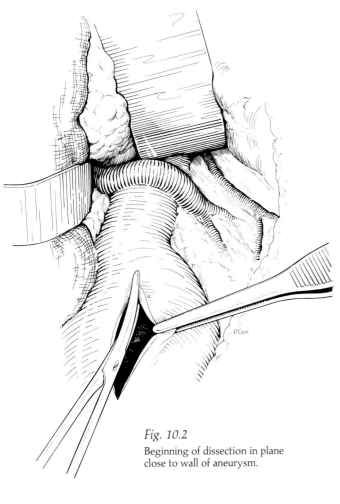

Fig. 10.2
Beginning of dissection in plane
close to wall of aneurysm.

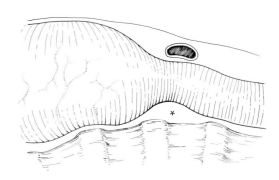

Fig. 10.3
Lateral view of neck showing thickening of periaortic
tissues as renal vein is approached from below
window behind neck.

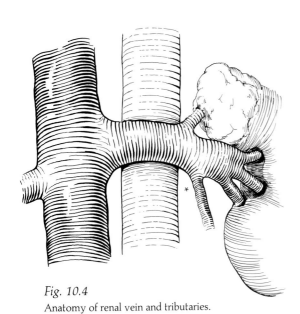

Fig. 10.4
Anatomy of renal vein and tributaries.

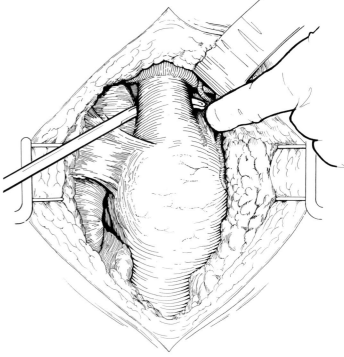

Fig. 10.5
Clamp being passed around aorta.

Attention is now turned to the area of the aortic bifurcation. The upper retractors are relaxed. The incision through the peritoneum inferior to the duodenum is continued inferiorly in the area between the aorta and the inferior vena cava, down over the aortic bifurcation and the right common iliac artery (Fig. 10.6). This technique minimizes damage to the autonomic nerves which are in the tissue in front of the aorta and its bifurcation. Preservation of these nerves reduces the chances of sexual dysfunction (particularly retrograde ejaculation) following aortic surgery. If the iliac artery is not aneurysmal, the dissection may stop short of the iliac bifurcation. If the common iliac artery is to be bypassed, the dissection should continue to the external iliac artery. The right ureter should be identified crossing the bifurcation of the common iliac artery. It is best avoided if the dissection is as close as possible to the wall of the artery and the tissues anterior to the artery are lifted forwards.

If the common iliac artery is to be used, it needs to be dissected to allow the safe application of a clamp. Dissection is carried out lateral and medial to the artery. This is one of the most dangerous parts of the operation because of the proximity of the area where the common iliac veins join to form the inferior vena cava. It is often possible to lift the artery forwards with fingers or forceps, to open up the plane behind the artery in front of the veins. It is not essential to encircle the artery at this point: sufficient dissection to allow the application of a clamp across the artery *and* knowledge of the position of the veins is all that is required. (For the management of vein injuries in this site see p. 174.)

The left common iliac artery is now dissected. In female patients the anterior wall of the left common iliac artery can be approached directly. In the dissection to preserve the autonomic nerves in male patients, a flap of retroperitoneal tissue containing the nerves is raised across the front of the aortic bifurcation to the left common iliac artery. Sometimes the exposure of the artery is inadequate with this approach. In these cases the artery can be approached directly, as in female patients, or the distal common iliac artery can be approached in the root of the sigmoid mesentery (Fig. 10.7). Dissection begins in the line of fusion between the peritoneal layers in the left paracolic gutter. As the sigmoid colon is mobilized medially, the external iliac artery can be seen and palpated. The left ureter lies in the base of the mesentery and should be positively identified as the iliac bifurcation is approached. Further mobilization of the retroperitoneal structures will display the left common iliac artery, which is dissected as described for the right common iliac artery. (This lateral approach to the iliac bifurcation is preferred if the external and internal iliac arteries are to be controlled. The steps for the further dissection of these arteries are discussed on p. 135.)

Application of clamps

Heparin 5000 units is given intravenously. After notifying the anaesthetist, clamps are applied (Fig. 10.8). Application of the clamps to the iliac arteries first reduces the chances of embolism ('trash') to the distal vessels. The clamps to be used are a matter of individual choice. It is simpler to place a clamp vertically across the aorta and this method is preferred in ruptured aneurysms. With the clamp in this position it may be difficult to suture the graft in the midline posteriorly. For this reason many prefer to apply a clamp transversely across the aorta. Application of the aortic clamp may be difficult, because it is often hard to find the posterior window through which the posterior blade of the clamp must be directed. It is often necessary to make several attempts before the clamp is passed safely. The clamp should be inserted from right to left to avoid the inferior vena cava. Most right-handed surgeons will find it easier to insert the clamp from left to right. If this is done, the left index finger should be placed between the inferior vena cava and the emerging tip of the clamp. The jaws of the clamp are closed just sufficiently firmly to abolish the pulse in the aorta.

Additional fixed retractor blades are placed over packs to retract the duodenum upwards and to the right, and the transverse mesocolon upwards and slightly left.

Insertion of graft

The graft is inserted using the inlay technique, the development of which was one of the major advances in aortic surgery. This method avoids the time-consuming and bloody dissection necessary to remove the posterior wall of the aneurysm.

The aneurysm is opened vertically, initially with a scalpel and then with scissors. The incision (Fig. 10.8) stops short of the ends of the aneurysm. A plane is developed easily between the wall of the aneurysm and the mural thrombus, which is removed. There may be rapid bleeding from the lumbar arteries at this stage. A dry pack should be placed in the lumen of the aneurysm. Pressure is applied to the pack while the anterior dissection is carried to within 2–3 mm of the neck of the aneurysm and lateral extensions made for about half to two-thirds of the circumference of the aorta. It is not necessary to transect the aorta.

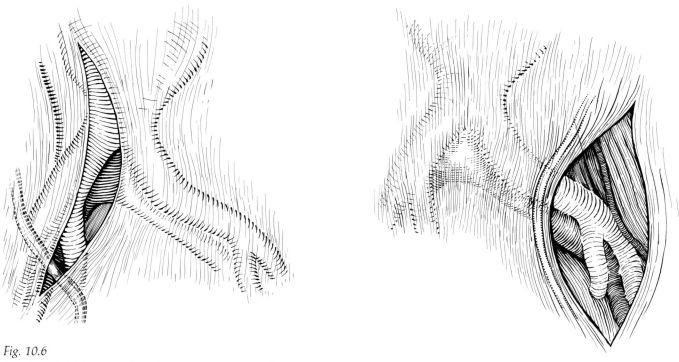

Fig. 10.6
Dissection of right common iliac artery.

Fig. 10.7
Dissection of left external iliac artery.

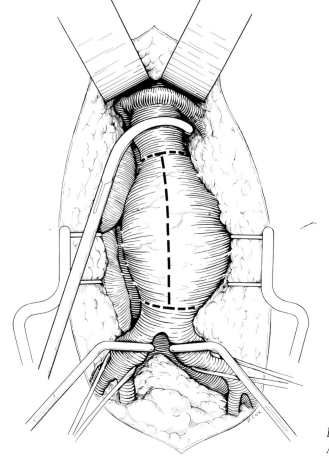

Fig. 10.8
Application of clamps and incision in aorta.

The pack is gradually withdrawn from proximal to distal and any bleeding lumbar arteries displayed sequentially. These are oversewn using 3/0 monofilament suture. If the orifices are surrounded by calcified plaque, this may be removed to allow the sutures to be placed in softer tissues. There may be vessels bleeding from the line of the neck of the aneurysm. If the bleeding is minor, these orifices can be incorporated in the posterior suture line. However, if there is significant bleeding, these vessels should be controlled at this stage to achieve optimal haemostasis before the insertion of the graft. The orifice of the inferior mesenteric artery should be sought close to the cut edge of the anterior wall of the aneurysm. If it is bleeding, it is oversewn. Reimplantation is necessary only in cases of demonstrated coeliac and superior mesenteric artery stenosis, or if the left colon is ischaemic at the conclusion of the operation. Perfect haemostasis provides optimal conditions of visibility and reduces the requirement for blood transfusion.

Proximal anastomosis
The graft to be used is selected. The majority of the grafts will be 18 or 20 mm in diameter. If a bifurcation graft is to be used, it should be cut transversely so that approximately 2 cm of the stem of the graft proximal to the bifurcation remains. The type of graft to be used is a matter of personal choice. The major choices are shown in Table 10.1. The decision may be influenced by availability and/or price.

Suture technique. There are a number of possible ways of suturing the proximal end of the graft. The anastomosis may be started at the corner or in the midline. The first suture may be tied or an open ('parachute') technique used. The preferred method is to start the anastomosis in the corner away from the surgeon and to tie down the first suture. The advantages of this are that

Table 10.1   Choice of graft

Material	Advantages	Disadvantages
Dacron		
Knitted Single or double Velour	Soft, easy to suture	Porosity, must be preclotted before administering heparin
Knitted Impregnated Gelatin Collagen	Low porosity	Stiffer than non-impregnated graft softer than woven graft
Woven	Low porosity Least well incorporated	Stiffest, passage of needles most difficult
PTFE		
	Low porosity Well incorporated	Moderately stiff Suture holes leak

all the suturing is performed towards the surgeon and, with the graft secured, it is easier to maintain tension so that the suture line does not leak because of loose sutures. With the parachute technique, it is easier to place the sutures; the first two or three may be quite difficult to place when the graft is tied down. However, it may be more difficult to achieve appropriate tension in the suture line when the parachute technique is used.

A double-ended 3/0 monofilament suture on an 18 mm needle is used. The first suture is placed as shown in Figure 10.9. It is placed at the posterior limit of the transverse incision at the level of the neck of the aneurysm. This will be at, or just behind, the mid-lateral point on the circumference of the aorta. It is important that distinct bites are taken of the aorta above the aneurysm and the wall of the aneurysm as shown. There should be a deliberate attempt to include as much of the wall of the aneurysm as possible in the suture line to give it added support against the sutures tearing through the wall of the aorta. The suture is tied securely. The knot is outside the graft and inside the lumen of the aneurysm. One of the needles is passed out of the field and secured.

The other needle is used for the posterior wall of the anastomosis. The graft is displaced up and towards the operator. The needle is passed into the luminal surface of the wall of the aneurysm (Fig. 10.10) and through the wall of the aorta into the lumen. The graft is returned to the floor of the aneurysmal sac and the suture is pulled gently into the lumen using a rotatory movement so that the needle does not tear the wall. The needle is then passed through the prosthesis from the luminal aspect (Fig. 10.11). In the same way succeeding sutures should attempt to incorporate the full thickness of the wall of the aneurysm as well as the full thickness of the wall of the aorta (see Fig. 10.12). Placement of the next one or two sutures may require the graft to be displaced in the manner described. Subsequently, it is usually possible to place a single bite through the luminal surface of the graft, the wall of the aneurysm and the wall of the aorta (Fig. 10.13).

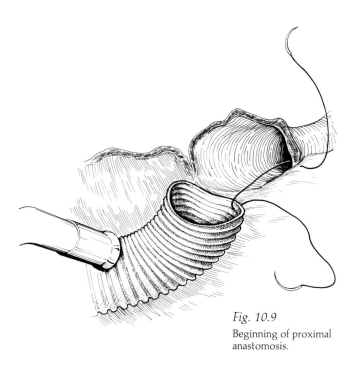

Fig. 10.9
Beginning of proximal
anastomosis.

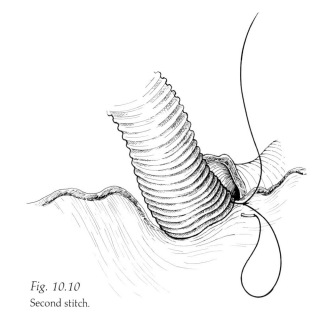

Fig. 10.10
Second stitch.

Fig. 10.12
Side view showing suture
through two layers of aorta.

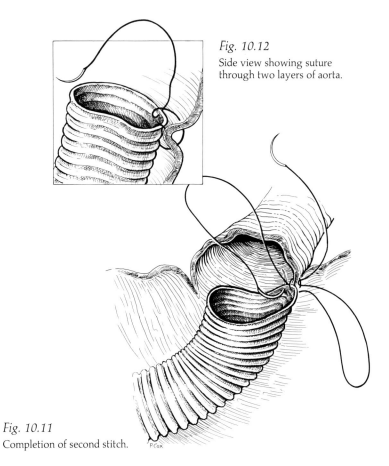

Fig. 10.11
Completion of second stitch.

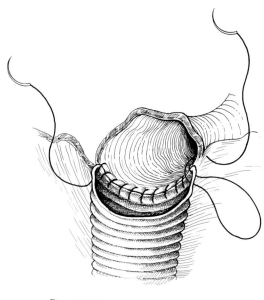

Fig. 10.13
Beginning of anterior wall.

Note that this technique is contrary to the conventional teaching that the needle should always be passed through an artery from its luminal surface to avoid lifting plaques which may then dissect and narrow the lumen. It is used in this situation because it is very difficult, unless the exposure is unusually good, to place the needle into the lumen of the aorta and retrieve it through the lumen of the graft. The ease with which thicker bites of the walls are obtained is a further advantage of the technique described.

The posterior wall of the anastomosis proceeds in this manner along the ridge which marks the neck of the aneurysm. If the neck is not clearly defined it is usually possible to create a neck using the technique described. An assistant should keep this suture under firm tension. Suturing should continue until the mid-lateral point has been reached. The last suture should pass through the graft so that it lies in the lumen of the aneurysm (Fig. 10.13).

The needle which was displaced from the wound after tying the first suture is now retrieved. It is passed through the wall of the graft from the outside and through the wall of the aorta from its luminal surface (Fig. 10.13). For the first two or three sutures, added support for the suture line can be obtained if the suture is then passed from outside the wall of the aneurysm into the lumen. Once the suture line comes around onto the anterior wall of the aorta, the tension with which the suture is held must lessen, in order to avoid the suture tearing through the aortic wall. If this pattern is continued, suturing reaches the first-used suture so that a knot can be tied neatly across the anastomosis. The ends are cut 1 cm long.

Testing the anastomosis. The anaesthetist should be informed when the anastomosis is about three-quarters

complete so that he/she may prepare to increase the rate of infusion should the anastomosis leak. When the final suture has been tied, the anastomosis is tested. A second clamp is placed across the graft about 1 cm distal to the anastomosis. The posterior wall of the anastomosis is inspected first because this is the commonest site of troublesome leaks. The graft is displaced proximally out of the wound and, after informing the anaesthetist, the proximal clamp is released for one or two heart beats.

The suture line is inspected and any significant leaks identified. The management of these is discussed on page 30. Any of the common patterns may be encountered. A larger area of bleeding is a serious problem. In the posterior wall, this usually results from failure to suture the full thickness of the wall of the aorta. It is treated by a continuous suture, taking bites as deep as possible across the leaking area (Fig. 10.14). In the anterior wall, the tear may result from placing the sutures too close together at the same depth: the effect is like tearing the perforations between stamps.

Haemorrhage from a torn lumbar artery behind the aorta may be particularly troublesome. It usually occurs in the region of the neck of the aneurysm and it may be impossible to see the site of the bleeding. Haemorrhage may be controlled temporarily by packing the area with a gauze swab, but removal of the swab is usually followed by recurrence of bleeding. The vessel may be controlled by more extensive mobilization of the posterolateral aspect of the aorta in the region of the bleeding. This manoeuvre, which is easier on the left side, may allow the site to be identified and controlled with a metal clip. If the bleeding is not controlled, the aorta should be transected distal to the neck of the

aneurysm, and the proximal segment lifted forwards until the site of bleeding is identified and controlled. If this is done before the proximal anastomosis has been completed, an end-to-end proximal anastomosis is performed. If the anastomosis has been sutured, the graft can be lifted forwards and the remaining posterior wall of the aneurysm divided distal to the suture line.

The operation must not proceed until haemostasis at the proximal anastomosis is secure. This particularly applies to the posterior wall, which is inaccessible once the lower anastomosis has been performed. Small areas of bleeding on the anterior wall may be left for later review. If achieving haemostasis is proving difficult, application of packs, carefully placed sequentially over the suture line and into the wound, may help. The top clamp is loosened and firm pressure applied to the packs for not less than 5 minutes, after which they are removed gently. Pleasant surprises often occur at this stage because the haemostatic mechanisms have been successful. Continued bleeding will probably require more sutures.

When haemostasis is secure, the lower clamp is removed and the blood is washed out of the graft using liberal amounts of heparinized saline solution.

The blades retracting the duodenum and mesocolon are relaxed and similar blades placed to retract the tissues on either side of the iliac arteries.

Lower anastomosis
The graft must first be cut to an appropriate length. A Dacron graft is cut while held under tension. If tension is not applied, the graft will elongate when arterial flow is restored and, because of the prominence of the graft pulse, the patient (and his physician) will be anxious that the aneurysm has

recurred. The graft should be cut
sufficiently short so that longitudinal
traction must be applied to the graft to
allow the initial sutures to be tied.

The same choices in suturing technique
are available as for the proximal
anastomosis. A method starting in the
midline posteriorly is illustrated in
Figure 10.15; the first suture has been
tied as described for the proximal
anastomosis. (In Figure 11.2 (p. 135) the
parachute technique is shown.) The
major difference from the proximal
anastomosis is that the sutures are
passed through the luminal surface of
the aortic bifurcation. This is because
exposure is better at the lower end, and
suturing is performed in a forehand
direction (for a right-handed surgeon
standing on the right side of the patient
or a left-handed surgeon standing on
the left).

There is frequently calcified plaque
around the aortic bifurcation. An
endarterectomy of this should not be
performed, because the plaque may
dissect into the iliac arteries and
predispose to occlusion. However, loose
fragments of atheroma may be trimmed
and removed. The technique for dealing
with calcified plaque is illustrated on
page 190. This part of the anastomosis
should be performed with great care to
avoid fracturing or dissecting the
plaque.

When the anastomosis is about three-
quarters complete the anaesthetist
should be advised and the vessels
flushed. The graft is flushed with
heparinized saline after releasing and
reapplying the proximal aortic clamp.
The orifice of each iliac artery is flushed
and the iliac clamps released in turn. The
clamps are reapplied and the blood
washed away with heparinized saline.
The anastomosis is completed.

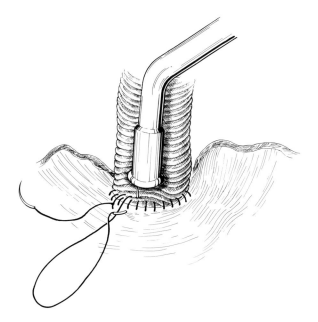

Fig. 10.14
Oversewing part of posterior wall.

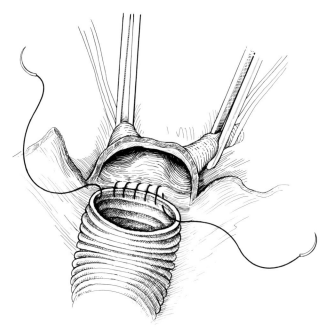

Fig. 10.15
Beginning of distal anastomosis.

Declamping

Air is expelled from the lumen by briefly releasing the aortic clamp. The lower anastomosis is inspected for leaks which, if present, are treated as described above. This is a critical stage of the procedure, particularly in patients with ruptured aneurysm. Declamping of the iliac arteries must be done carefully to avoid major instability of the circulation. The surgeon should be able to see the continuously monitored blood pressure tracing. The clamp is released from one of the iliac arteries and the vessel occluded between the surgeon's finger and thumb. Blood is allowed to flow into the iliac artery while the blood pressure tracing is inspected. Suddenly releasing the clamp will sometimes result in profound hypotension. The effects of this are worsened because the distribution of the blood flow is to the vasodilated limb and away from vital organs. If there is a fall in the systolic pressure of more than 20 mmHg or a fall of greater than 10 mmHg which lasts longer than 30 seconds, the artery should be occluded while the anaethetist infuses fluid intravenously. After a period of 3–5 minutes, the artery is released again and usually the blood pressure is more stable. This process may need to be repeated several times and, when the blood pressure is stable, it is repeated in the other limb. The presence of palpable femoral pulses is confirmed and, if the feet are exposed, they are inspected. If the superficial femoral artery is occluded, it may take hours for normal colour to return to the feet.

When the circulation is stable and haemostasis secure, the graft is covered by the wall of the aneurysm (Fig. 10.16). This is to prevent adhesion between the bowel (especially duodenum) and the graft, which may result in aortoduodenal fistula (see p. 227). This condition should be regarded as being preventable. Particular attention should be given to the region of the upper anastomosis where coverage of the graft by aneurysm wall may be more difficult. If necessary, greater omentum should be used to ensure that the graft is adequately separated from the duodenum.

Before replacing the small bowel within the abdominal cavity, the left colon should be inspected to ensure that it has an adequate blood supply. Colon ischaemia is usually multifactorial in origin. The common elements are interruption of the arterial supply and hypovolaemia. Preservation of internal iliac blood flow will lessen the effects of interruption of the inferior mesenteric artery. If there is concern about the adequacy of the blood supply, a sterile Doppler probe may be used to examine the vessels in the mesentery and on the wall of the colon (See Ernst 1983 for review). If there is doubt about the viability of the colon and the patient's circulation is unstable, the abdomen should be closed and colonoscopy or a second-look laparotomy performed in 8–12 hours. If it is necessary to reimplant the inferior mesenteric artery, one of the techniques used for reimplantation of the renal artery described on page 158 should be used.

The abdomen is closed in the usual fashion for wounds with a high risk of burst abdomen. A mass closure technique with continuous sutures of monofilament nylon or prolene is preferred.

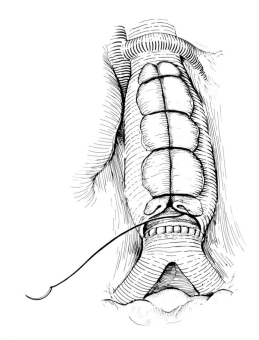

Fig. 10.16
Wall sutured over graft.

LOWER LIMB ISCHAEMIA

Prevention

The development of ischaemic feet can be a catastrophic consequence of aneurysm repair. Two common causes are technical problems with a distal anastomosis (commonly due to errors in suturing or damage at the site of application of the distal clamps) and embolism to a large artery (common femoral or popliteal). In addition there is a small group of patients who develop ischaemic feet despite the presence of ankle pulses. These are colloquially called 'trash feet' in recognition of the likely aetiology, which is embolism of the small arteries of the feet by material from the area of the operation. This may include the contents of the aneurysm or material from the region of application of the distal clamps. The prevention of this problem has been detailed most carefully by Imparato (1983). He described the following sequence to the dissection:

1. Dissect the external and internal iliac arteries on each side.
2. Dissect the lower border of the left renal vein as described above.
3. Administer heparin as soon as it is clear that it will be possible to place an infrarenal clamp on the aorta.
4. Clamp the external and internal iliac arteries in turn on each side.
5. Complete dissection of the neck of the aneurysm and perform the proximal anastomosis.
6. Bifurcation grafts are almost always used.
7. The right limb of the graft is anastomosed to the distal right common iliac artery as described.
8. If back-bleeding from the external iliac artery is sparse, a rubber catheter (not a balloon catheter) is passed distally to open the artery at the site of the clamp. Irrigate the lumen and complete the anastomosis.

9. Flush the graft with 25–50 ml blood by releasing the aortic clamp. Irrigate the graft and repeat the procedure until there is no longer any clot or atheromatous debris present.
10. Restore flow first to the internal and then to the external iliac artery.
11. Perform the left anastomosis in similar fashion.

Review of the published accounts of techniques for aneurysm repair suggests that, while most authors are conscious of the problem of lower limb ischaemia, they do not adopt such elaborate routines to prevent it.

Treatment

Loss of femoral pulse(s)
If a femoral pulse does not return, the femoral artery should be opened distal to the inguinal ligament and a balloon catheter passed proximally into the graft. The position of the balloon should be palpated carefully. Withdrawal of the catheter usually results in profuse flow whereupon the femoral artery can be closed after irrigation to remove any loose pieces of atheroma or thrombus. If the flow is still inadequate, it is likely to be due to an anastomotic stenosis which should be revised, or occlusive disease distally in the external iliac artery. In this case a prosthetic bypass graft should be inserted from the aortic graft to the common femoral artery.

Loss of distal pulses
An angiogram should be performed via the femoral artery as described on page 13. If the popliteal pulse has been lost, the likely causes are embolus, thrombosis of a popliteal aneurysm or occlusion of a diseased superficial femoral artery. Each of these conditions should be treated as required.

Loss of one ankle pulse can be ignored if perfusion of the foot is satisfactory. If both ankle pulses are lost, popliteal occlusion should be suspected.

Ischaemic feet with palpable ankle pulses
Passage of balloon catheters should be avoided because occlusions are in vessels which cannot be cleared with a balloon catheter. Measures to prevent propagation of thrombus, such as heparin or low-molecular-weight dextran, should be used. There is probably nothing else which can be done to change the outcome of this condition.

POSTOPERATIVE CARE

The after-care required for these patients is described on page 19.

RESULTS OF ELECTIVE SURGERY

More than 95% of patients undergoing elective operation will survive the procedure. Excellent results have been reported in series of elderly patients (O'Donnell et al 1976), and patients regarded as being at high risk because of the presence of severe cardiac, respiratory or renal disease (Hollier 1986). Many centres have reported a higher mortality (10–15%) in patients who undergo urgent operation for symptoms of impending rupture but in whom the aneurysm is not ruptured.

Following surgery the life expectancy of patients approaches normal. The difference between the aneurysm and control subjects is probably due to the higher prevalence of coronary artery disease in the former group.

REFERENCES

Cabellon S, Moncreif C L, Pierre D R, Cavanaugh D G 1983 Incidence of abdominal aortic aneurysm in patients with atheromatous arterial disease. American Journal of Surgery 146: 575–576

Castleden W M, Mercer J C and Members of the Western Australian Vascular Service 1985 Abdominal aortic aneurysms in Western Australia: descriptive epidemiology and patterns of rupture. British Journal of Surgery 72: 109–112

Collin J, Araujo L, Walton J, Lindsell D 1988 Oxford screening programme for abdominal aortic aneurysms in men aged 65 to 74 years. Lancet ii: 613–615

Ernst C B 1983 Prevention of intestinal ischaemia following abdominal aortic reconstruction. Surgery 93: 102–106

Hollier L H 1986 Surgical management of abdominal aortic aneurysm in the high-risk patient. Surgical Clinics of North America 66: 269–279

Imparato A M 1983 Abdominal aortic surgery: prevention of lower limb ischaemia. Surgery 93: 112–116

O'Donnell T F, Darling R C, Linton R R 1976 Is 80 years too old for aneurysmectomy? Archives of Surgery 111: 1250–1257

Thomas P R S, Stewart R D 1988 Abdominal aortic aneurysm. British Journal of Surgery 75: 733–736

Thurmond A 1986 Abdominal aortic aneurysm: incidence in a population at risk. Journal of Cardiovascular Surgery 27: 457–459

Todd G J, Nowygrod R, Benvenisty A, Buda J, Reetsma K 1991 The accuracy of CT scanning in the diagnosis of abdominal and thoracoabdominal aortic aneurysms. Journal of Vascular Surgery 13: 302–310

Webster M W, St Jean P L, Steed D L, Ferrell R E, Majumder P P 1991 Abdominal aortic aneurysm: results of a family study. Journal of Vascular Surgery 13: 366–372

Chapter 11

Alternative techniques

INCISIONS

1.   Retroperitoneal approach (see p. 109).
2.   Bilateral subcostal incision (Fig. 11.1).

This incision crosses the midline midway between the xiphoid process and the umbilicus. On each side, the incision is curved inferiorly and extends for about 10–15 cm on each side, passing 5 cm beneath the costal margin. The subcutaneous tissue and the anterior rectus sheath are incised. The rectus muscles are divided with diathermy. Lateral to the rectus sheath, the external oblique muscle is divided and the other muscles split. The peritoneal cavity is opened by incising the posterior rectus sheath. The falciform ligament is divided between clamps. The blades of a self-retaining retractor are placed in the midline and the small bowel lies over the right corner of the wound. The incision is closed in layers using continuous, monofilament, non-absorbable sutures.

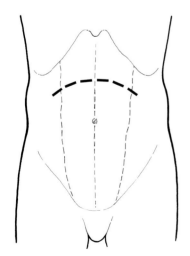

Fig. 11.1
Subcostal incision.

This incision gives excellent access to the region of the renal arteries. However, it takes longer than a midline incision, there is more bleeding from the wound and access to the distal iliac arteries may be difficult.

VARIATIONS IN ANASTOMOSIS

Proximal

Parachute technique
In this technique, a number of sutures are placed before any of them are tightened (see fig. 11.2). The technique works best with monofilament nylon or polypropylene sutures, but it is possible, although more difficult, with polytetrafluoroethylene (PTFE) sutures. In the aortic anastomosis being considered, this may involve most or all of the posterior wall. The sutures are placed as shown in the figure and are tightened by traction on both ends of the suture and the graft. Pulling the sutures alone will result in least tension in the centre of the suture line. The graft is moved in a to-and-fro motion and this manoeuvre results in more even distribution of tension. Once the aorta and graft have been brought together, the graft is lifted forwards so that the suture line can be inspected from outside the anastomosis. Further tightening of the suture can be achieved by passing a nerve (sympathectomy) hook beneath loose threads, and progressively tightening the suture towards one end of the anastomosis. The advantage of this technique is that it is easier to place sutures precisely. For this reason, this technique is used when anastomosing small vessels. However, in the aorta, such precise suture placement is not critical and the importance of ensuring adequate thickness of tissue has been emphasized in the account of the suturing technique given above. In addition, it may be difficult to tighten the suture and excessive traction may cause tearing of the aortic wall.

Suturing from the middle of the posterior wall
This technique is used by many experienced surgeons and is described for the distal aortic anastomosis. Starting the anastomosis from the side facilitates the formation of the ridge along the posterior wall, and this enables greater certainty in ensuring that the sutures pass through both the aneurysm and the wall of the aorta as shown in Figure 10.12.

LOWER END PROBLEMS

Straight or bifurcated graft?
The major decision which needs to be taken is whether to use a straight or a bifurcated graft. This decision will depend on the presence of occlusive disease in the iliac vessels and the state of the aortic bifurcation. If iliac occlusion is a significant problem, a conventional aortobifemoral graft should be placed with the distal anastomosis on the common femoral artery.

In about 80% of patients with aortic aneurysm, a straight graft can be used. The region of the bifurcation is inspected. If a graft which is suitable for the proximal aorta can be sutured around the aortic bifurcation, and neither common iliac artery is more than 2 cm in diameter, a straight graft is used. If the aortic bifurcation is clearly aneurysmal, a bifurcation graft should be used. The decision is sometimes difficult. If a straight graft can be used the operation is quicker and less dissection is required. However, iliac aneurysms can expand and rupture although this is an infrequent event. A straight graft is used whenever it is technically possible to do so and the risks associated with leaving mildly dilated iliac arteries are accepted.

If the circumference of the lower aorta is greater than that of the graft, one of two manoeuvres may be used.

1. A broad 'V' is cut in the distal end of the graft (Gilling-Smith & Wolfe 1986). This provides an increase in the circumference of the lower end of the graft and allows the suturing of the lower anastomosis without tension (Fig. 11.3). The apex of the 'V' corresponds to the length of graft required.

2. A cut 1 cm long can be made in the anterior midline of the graft and the corners trimmed. This technique is useful if disproportion becomes obvious as the anastomosis is being completed. A longer incision may result in tearing of the wall of the aorta as a result of excessive tension.

Iliac anastomoses

It is important to maintain blood flow to the pelvic viscera, including the sigmoid colon, by maintaining flow to at least one internal iliac artery. This factor may determine which of the techniques described may be used.

Exposure

If an iliac anastomosis is to be peformed, other than to the orifice of the common iliac artery, the external and internal iliac arteries must be controlled.

On the right side this can be performed by continuing the dissection of the common iliac artery distally, beyond its bifurcation. The dissection is kept close to the wall of the artery to avoid damaging the ureter. The ureter should always be positively identified and can be displaced safely from the vessels. It is usually possible to obtain a sufficent length of external iliac artery because the dissection can be continued laterally to the ureter, down to the inguinal ligament if necessary. The external iliac artery can usually be elevated in the fingers and then encircled with a tape.

The internal iliac is sought by palpation below the point where the common iliac artery decreases in diameter. The trunk of the artery is carefully dissected, avoiding trauma to the vein which lies deep to the artery. It is not necessary to encircle the artery.

On the left side, the dissection is conducted on both sides of the sigmoid mesentery, in the base of which the ureter is situated as described above. The external iliac artery is dissected from the lateral side of the mesentery. The internal iliac artery is dissected in a similar manner from the right side.

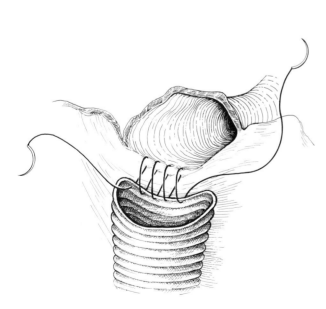

Fig. 11.2
Parachute technique.

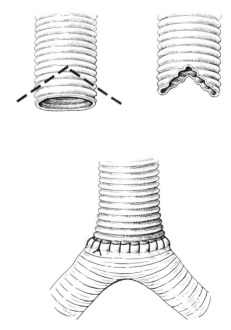

Fig. 11.3
Method of widening lower end of graft.

Anastomosis to orifice of common iliac artery

If one iliac orifice and ipsilateral common iliac artery are normal, a limb of the bifurcation graft can be sutured to this orifice (Fig. 11.4). The contralateral internal iliac artery need not be preserved.

Distal iliac anastomoses

There are two methods of performing the iliac anastomosis which will preserve flow in the internal iliac artery.

1.   The method used most commonly is to open the common iliac artery distally until the orifices of the internal and external iliac arteries can be seen. The limb of the graft is cut obliquely and sutured around both orifices, restoring blood flow to them both (Fig. 11.5a–c).

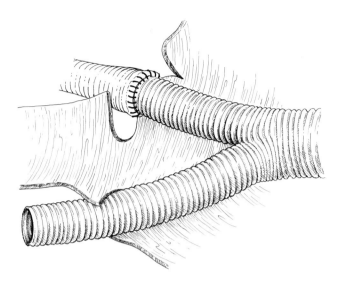

Fig. 11.4
Anastomosis to origin of common iliac artery.

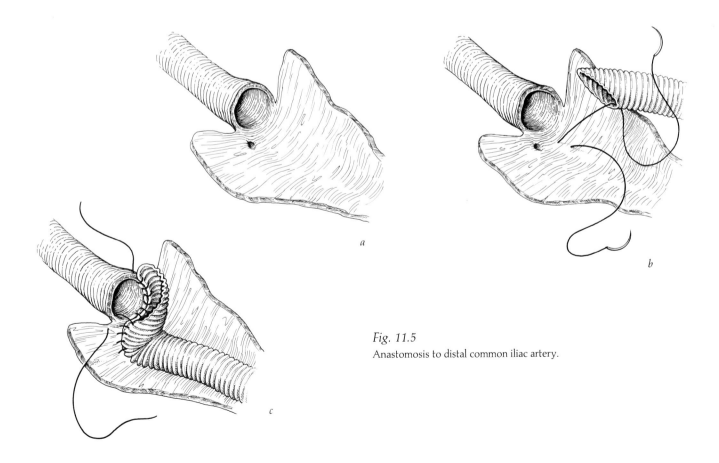

Fig. 11.5
Anastomosis to distal common iliac artery.

2. The distal common iliac artery can be occluded by ligatures or by the application of a row of staples across it (Fig. 11.6). Application of ligatures may be difficult because of the large diameter of the vessel. A longitudinal incision is then made in a convenient part of the external iliac artery, and an anastomosis fashioned between the end of the graft and the side of the artery.

If the internal iliac artery is not to be preserved, the external iliac artery is transected distal to a ligature and an end-to-end anastomosis is performed (Fig. 11.7). This is the easiest procedure because the anastomosis can be performed in the superficial parts of the wound. In this case, the graft is brought over the surface of the common iliac artery, behind the ureter, in the same retroperitoneal plane as for an aortofemoral graft. The orifice of the common iliac artery must be obliterated from within the aneurysm to control blood loss from back-bleeding from the internal iliac artery.

The iliac limbs of the graft are brought through the former lumen of the common iliac arteries and can be covered by suturing the artery wall over them.

NON-SUTURED GRAFT

There were several early attempts to perform vascular anastomoses without direct suture of the ends of the vessel. Many of these involved using a prosthetic metal tube or methods where one end of the vessel was invaginated in the other end. These methods were discarded following the work of Carrel and Guthrie, who described the technique for performing a sutured anastomosis, the principles of which are still applied in modern techniques.

There are several situations in the surgery of aortic aneurysm where the conventional techniques may be difficult to apply. The most important of these is acute dissection of the aorta (Chapter 7) where the friability of the aortic wall may cause difficult technical problems because of the tendency of sutures to tear out of the tissue. In other patients the greatest dilatation of the aorta may be infrarenal but ectasia of the aorta may make it difficult to define a neck for suturing. In these cases the intraluminal prosthesis may have a place. Its use has also been advocated in thoracic aneurysms because the anastomosis can be performed faster than a sutured anastomosis.

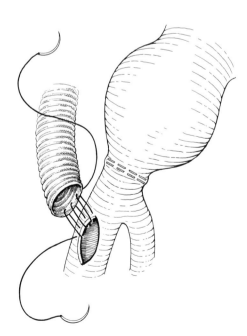

Fig. 11.6
Anastomosis to external iliac artery: end-to-side.

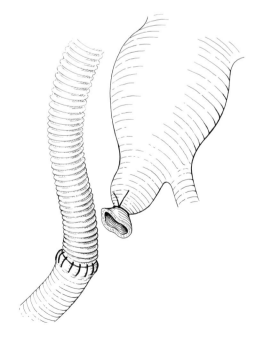

Fig. 11.7
Anastomosis to external iliac artery: end-to-end.

The prosthesis

The commercially available prosthesis consists of a tube of woven Dacron, 20 or 22 mm in diameter (Fig. 11.8). Attached to the proximal end is a rigid ring 10 mm wide which has a shallow groove. A similar ring can be moved up and down the graft so that the graft can be cut to a suitable length.

Technique

The aorta is dissected as described on page 122 and a Dacron tape 4 mm wide placed around it in the position of the upper end of the graft. The prosthesis is inserted into the aorta and the tape tied so that it lies in the groove in the ring on the graft. The insertion of the prosthesis is aided by using a device such as that described by Harris (1990), which comprises a Travers retractor modified by the removal of the teeth so that the end is a flat flange which is inserted between the ring and the Dacron tube. In this way the graft can be pushed up into the aorta. The tape must be tied tightly around the ring. It is essential that the graft chosen not be too wide. Forcible attempts to insert the prosthesis may cause serious damage to the vessel wall. The ring on the prosthesis reduces the diameter of the tube graft by about 4 mm. Thus it is recommended that the technique not be used unless the internal diameter of the aorta is at least 20 mm. In order to guard against displacement or tilting of the prosthesis, two methods may be used to secure the prosthesis. A second tape may be tied around the aorta so that it lies just distal to the ring on the prosthesis (Fig. 11.9). Alternatively, sutures may be placed between the wall of the aorta and the prosthesis to fix it more securely. An additional problem is that the aortic clamp must be placed more proximally than normal to allow room for the insertion of the graft. Thus it is usually impossible to apply an infrarenal clamp in patients with abdominal aortic aneurysm. In these cases, the aorta may be controlled by an intraluminal balloon or a suprarenal clamp. These constraints mean that the technique will be suitable only rarely in patients with abdominal aortic aneurysm.

The distal anastomoses are performed in the routine manner. The sutureless technique may be applied. The graft is cut to the appropriate length, the lower ring is placed over the end of the graft, which is inserted into the aorta and secured by tying a tape to fit in the lower ring.

Outcomes

There are several reports of the use of these prostheses in thoracic aneurysms or dissections (Koyamada et al 1985). Harris (1990) has reported good results when used in patients with thoracoabdominal aneurysm. The ease of performance of the proximal anastomosis seems to be confirmed by these reports and there seem to be few complications specific to these devices.

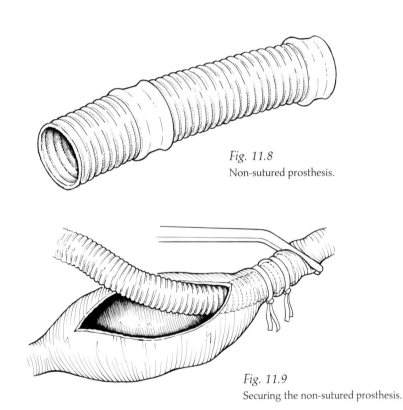

Fig. 11.8
Non-sutured prosthesis.

Fig. 11.9
Securing the non-sutured prosthesis.

REFERENCES

Gilling-Smith G L, Wolfe J H N 1986 The tailed aortic graft: a technique for widening the distal orifice of an aortic tube graft. British Journal of Surgery 73: 208
Harris P L 1990 An intraluminal non-sutured graft for aortic aneurysm repairs. In: Greenhalgh R M, Mannick J A, Powell J T (eds) The cause and management of aneurysms. W B Saunders, London, pp 401–408
Koyamada K, Ishikawa S, Yamaki S, Kakihata H 1985 Surgical treatment for dissecting aneurysm of the aorta using a double ringed graft. Journal of Cardiovascular Surgery 26: 488–491

Chapter 12

Ruptured abdominal aortic aneurysm

Introduction

This remains one of the most dramatic conditions encountered in vascular surgery and its incidence appears to be increasing. Data from community surveys suggest that the overall mortality of this condition is of the order of 80%, with the survival of patients in whom resection is undertaken being in the range of 50–60% (Ingoldby et al 1986, Johansen et al 1991). There is disturbing evidence that aggressive pre-hospital care results in the arrival in hospital of many patients who are destined to die (Johansen et al 1991). Some tertiary referral centres are able to produce better results following operation. One reason may be that they receive a selected group of patients who are able to survive the time and distance necessary to transfer them to the institution where surgery is to be performed.

In most patients who present with ruptured aneurysm, this is the first manifestation of the disease. There has been interest in recent years in the possibility that screening of asymptomatic patients may be able to reduce the mortality from rupture. There is reasonable evidence that the cost of screening all males between the ages of 65 and 74 years would be of the order of £9000 per life saved (Collin 1985).

CLINICAL FEATURES

There is a wide variation in the severity of the onset of rupture. Some patients collapse and die rapidly. At the other extreme patients may present with a contained rupture which may remain stable for days or weeks. The triad of back pain, hypovolaemia and a palpable aneurysm is diagnostic. However, up to 30% of patients are not diagnosed at the time of admission to hospital. The commonest misdiagnosis is to label the patient as having ureteric colic. Fortunately, this may not be too serious, because, if an urgent intravenous urogram is performed, signs of an aneurysm or ureteric displacement by haematoma may allow the diagnosis to be made with minimal delay. Difficulties arise in the 30% of patients in whom the aneurysm is not easily palpable. These include obese patients and patients with a small aneurysm. If hypovolaemia is not prominent, the diagnosis may not be made for several days until further bleeding occurs.

INDICATIONS FOR OPERATION

Very few patients with ruptured abdominal aortic aneurysm survive without operation. Thus all patients in whom the diagnosis is made should be considered for surgery. However, operation is not advised in the presence of disseminated malignant disease or severe cerebrovascular disease. It should be emphasized that, because of the urgency of the situation, detailed information about the patient's premorbid condition may be unavailable and, in these circumstances, the surgeon is obliged to undertake laparotomy.

Evidence is accumulating about the factors which adversely affect the outlook in these patients. For example, it is suggested that a patient who suffers a cardiac arrest before arrival in the operating theatre, or a female patient, aged 80 years or more who is profoundly shocked, has a very small chance of surviving operation. It may be appropriate in these circumstances not to undertake operation.

PREOPERATIVE PREPARATION

The speed with which surgery must be undertaken depends on the haemodynamic status of the patient and this is a major determinant of survival. A patient in whom the diagnosis is clear or who is haemodynamically unstable must be transferred to the operating theatre at the earliest opportunity. The reason is that application of a clamp to the aorta is essential to allow resuscitation to proceed. The minimum time should be spent in preparing the patient by the insertion of vascular access lines and urinary catheter. It is a serious error to attempt to raise the blood pressure towards normal before the aortic clamp is applied: a blood pressure of 50–70 mmHg systolic is acceptable at this time (Crawford 1991). What often happens is that an attempt is made to raise the systolic blood pressure from 60 mmHg towards 100 mmHg. The blood pressure may rise following intravenous infusion of blood but, too frequently, this is followed by a catastrophic, and frequently fatal, fall in blood pressure as the raised blood pressure results in renewed intra-abdominal bleeding.

During the preparation of the patient the skin should be shaved and prepared and the drapes placed before the induction of anaesthesia. This is to minimize the time of any decompensation of the circulation before the aortic clamp is applied.

In less urgent cases, a more measured preparation may be undertaken but early transfer to the operating theatre is mandatory so that operation can be undertaken immediately signs of hypovolaemia appear. A rectal examination should be performed to ensure that gastrointestinal bleeding is not the cause of the hypovolaemia.

Preparations are made to set up the autotransfusion equipment if this is available, and the blood bank warned that platelet transfusion and fresh frozen plasma may be required (see p. 20).

INVESTIGATIONS

Blood is drawn for baseline haematology and biochemistry and for blood grouping and cross-matching. ECG should be performed to exclude myocardial infarction. Ischaemic changes may result from hypovolaemia. Further investigations, other than a chest radiograph to check the position of a central venous catheter, are inappropriate in most patients.

If the diagnosis is in doubt *and* the patient is haemodynamically stable, computed tomographic (CT) scanning should be performed (Johnson et al 1986, Kvilekval et al 1990). This procedure has a number of advantages:

1. The sensitivity of this investigation in diagnosing ruptured abdominal aortic aneurysm is close to 100%.
2. Other causes for the clinical presentation are identified in about 20% of patients.

3. Additional information which may affect operative management, such as the presence of vein anomalies, the presence of a horseshoe kidney or suprarenal extension of the aneurysm, is identified in about 25% of cases.

The reason for attempting to make a positive diagnosis of rupture, even when an aneurysm is palpable, is that emergency operation for unruptured aneurysm carries a mortality which is several times greater than for elective aneurysm. The reasons for this are not clear, but time spent in a careful, but expeditious, preparation of the patient for the next available elective operating list would be expected to reduce the mortality in these cases. Particular attention should be paid to the assessment of cardiopulmonary and renal function.

A member of the surgical team must remain in close attendance during the performance of the CT scan, which must be aborted should signs of hypovolaemia appear.

OPERATION

A long midline incision is used. No attempt is made to achieve haemostasis in the wound at this stage. The peritoneum is opened and the large retroperitoneal haematoma is usually obvious. There is frequently a small amount of heavily blood-stained peritoneal fluid, but free intraperitoneal blood is a bad prognostic sign.

The small bowel is eviscerated to the right side of the wound, and the transverse mesocolon and the greater omentum lifted out of the proximal part of the wound as for elective aneurysm (p. 122).

Controlling the aorta

The events of the next 2–5 minutes may determine the outcome of the operation. The essential step is to place a clamp across the aorta above the aneurysm. There are several ways of performing this manoeuvre.

The most effective is to place the clamp across the neck of the aneurysm on the infrarenal aorta. The steps in performing this are:

1.   Cut with scissors through the peritoneum to the left of the duodenum (Fig. 12.1). The duodenum is usually lifted up by the haematoma so that, once the peritoneum has been divided, the remainder of the dissection can be performed with fingers.
2.   Incise the haematoma over the region of the neck of the aneurysm. The bleeding usually remains contained at this stage.
3.   Burrow with the fingers into the haematoma until the aorta is felt. Continue the dissection with fingers until the vertebral column can be felt on each side of the aorta.
4.   Occlude the aorta by squeezing between thumb and fingers.
5.   With the occluding fingers in position, place a large straight aortic clamp vertically over the occluding hand until the tips are felt to contact the vertebral column (Fig. 12.2).
6.   Close the clamp and remove the hand which has been occluding the aorta. The aneurysm should not be pulsating.
7.   Check the position of the clamp by reinserting the fingers. It is most important that the clamp be against the vertebral column.

This is the fastest way of achieving control of the aorta. The dissection with the fingers is usually atraumatic. However, it is difficult to be certain of the exact position of the clamp, which may be placed, inadvertently, above the renal arteries and/or across the left renal vein. Sometimes tributaries of the renal vein are avulsed. These are minor difficulties compared with the need to clamp the aorta as quickly as possible.

Other methods of controlling the aorta
One of the oldest instruments in the vascular surgery pack is a device to compress the aorta before a clamp is applied. This may either be a wooden spoon with its bowl cut so that the end is concave or a metal instrument with a handle and a curved blade 10–15 mm wide and 3–4 cm long. Such a device may be used, but if the method described is employed it is seldom needed.

Supracoeliac clamping. This method is advocated by a number of experienced surgeons for temporary (Veith et al 1990) or definitive (Crawford 1991) control of the aorta. The aorta is dissected and clamped as it enters the abdomen through the diaphragm. The anatomy of the diaphragmatic crura and the aorta are shown in Figure 12.3a, b.

1.   Draw the stomach inferiorly and divide the lesser omentum.
2.   Feel for the aorta as it emerges through the diaphragm.
3.   Divide the posterior peritoneum by blunt or sharp dissection and incise the left crus vertically and develop the plane of dissection close to the aorta. At this point the periaortic tissues are loose and the aortic wall soft.
4.   No attempt should be made to dissect the posterior aspect of the aorta.
5.   Place fingers on either side of the aorta as described in the preceding section and apply a vertical clamp to the aorta.

This method has several disadvantages. First, access is not always easy in a large patient. Second, back-bleeding will still occur from the visceral and renal arteries. Third, the infrarenal dissection still has to be performed. Despite these reservations, this method is employed by many experienced surgeons to provide life-saving, temporary control of the aorta. Many would reposition the clamp to the infrarenal aorta before proceeding to the proximal anastomosis, although Crawford (1991) describes performing this anastomosis with the supracoeliac clamp in place and transferring the clamp to the graft after the anastomosis has been completed.

If access to the neck of the aneurysm is likely to be difficult, for example as a result of previous intra-abdominal sepsis or colonic or gastric surgery, a left anterolateral thoracotomy can be performed, and, after mobilizing the intrathoracic aorta, a clamp placed across it.

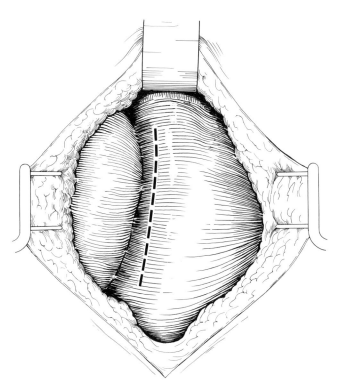

Fig. 12.1
Incision in retroperitoneal tissues.

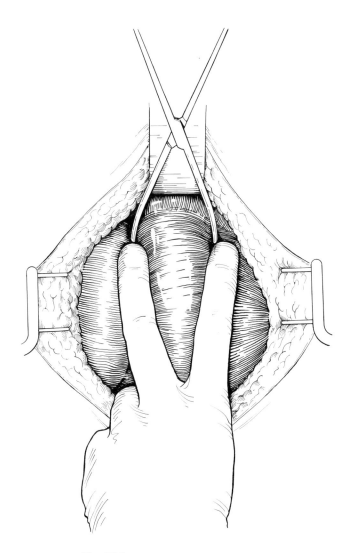

Fig. 12.2
Position of hand and application of clamp.

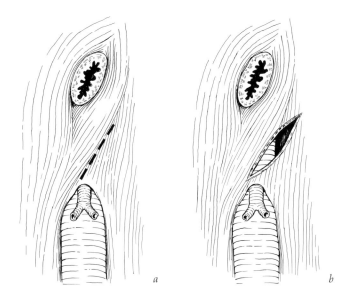

Fig. 12.3
Supracoeliac clamping—anatomy of crura—incision in left crus.

Use of balloon catheters. Two techniques have been described:

1. If there is free rupture of the aorta when the abdomen is opened, compress the suprarenal aorta and insert a Foley balloon catheter with a 30 ml balloon through the rent in the aortic wall into the suprarenal aorta.
2. Pass a balloon catheter through a cutdown in a brachial artery. Partially inflate the balloon once the aorta has been entered and there is easy passage into the descending aorta. Fully inflate the balloon when it is judged to be in the region of the diaphragm.

Iliac arteries

The peritoneum over the iliac arteries is incised and the fingers inserted through the haematoma until the iliac arteries are felt. These are grasped in turn between finger and thumb and a clamp applied. The tips of these clamps should be directed distally away from the aortic bifurcation and the confluence of the common iliac veins, to avoid damage to the veins.

Consolidation

Once the three clamps have been applied, the surgeon should pause, place packs in the wound and wait while the anaesthetist restores the circulating blood volume. The time elapsed since the skin incision is commonly about 5 minutes, compared with 30–45 minutes to reach the comparable stage in an elective operation.

At this stage, continuing blood loss should be minimal. The most serious cause is that the aortic clamp has not completely occluded the aorta. The usual reason for this is that the clamp has not been applied deeply enough against the vertebral column. The position may be helped by pushing the handles of the clamp to apply pressure against the vertebral column while the exploring hand is reinserted and the position of the clamp adjusted. Other

sources of arterial bleeding include the lumbar arteries, incompletely applied iliac artery clamps, or back-bleeding from visceral arteries if a supracoeliac clamp has been used. These are seldom a source of serious concern at this stage. Venous bleeding is more common and usually comes from the renal vein or its tributaries. Blood escaping from the retroperitoneal haematoma may continue to seep into the wound. This is not a major problem (apart from obscuring visibility), because it does not represent continuing loss from the circulation.

The next step is to place the aortic clamp in an optimal position to facilitate insertion of the graft. The haematoma over the proximal part of the anterior wall of the aneurysm is divided until the wall can be seen. The dissection is continued proximally until the region of the clamp and left renal vein is reached. The area of the application of the clamp is inspected and the renal arteries sought by palpation. If the clamp has been applied above one or both renal arteries or the left renal vein, it is repositioned appropriately. Usually the operation proceeds with the vertical clamp in position. However, if desired, a transverse clamp across the aorta can be placed at this stage. As mentioned above, some authors perform the proximal anastomosis with the supracoeliac clamp in place.

If tributaries have been avulsed from the left renal vein, they are ligated and the renal vein repaired. The inferior mesenteric vein may have been damaged. It is ligated if bleeding. Clamps can be applied to the left renal vein to control the bleeding. When this has been done holes in the vein can be sutured precisely, without continuing blood loss. (For the technique of repair of these tears see p. 173.)

This period of consolidation is important in the conduct of the

operation. It allows the surgeon and assistants temporary relaxation, and provides time for the anaesthetist to restore the circulating blood volume. Making haemostasis as good as possible facilitates the remainder of the operation by reducing the need for suction. Reduction of blood loss reduces the requirement for blood transfusion and the chances of developing coagulopathy due to loss of clotting factors. These are highly desirable objectives. From this point, blood loss should be no greater than in an elective operation.

Heparin 5000 units may be given intravenously at this stage, as in an elective operation, to prevent thrombosis in the static arterial system in the lower limbs. This is not an essential step. Alternatively, each iliac clamp may be removed in turn and, after removal of any clot or loose debris, 50–100 ml of heparinized saline solution injected.

Anastomoses

The aneurysm is opened and any thrombus removed. The site of rupture can be felt. This site may vary but is commonly posterolateral. If it is close to the neck it may reduce the amount of suitable tissue to which the graft may be sutured. Lumbar vessels are oversewn as in an elective operation.

The graft is inserted as in an elective operation (see p. 124). A porous graft should not be used because of the inability to preclot the graft.

POSTOPERATIVE CARE

Continued close monitoring of the circulation is critical in the early postoperative period. If the circulation remains stable for 6–8 hours the surgeon can be assured that haemostasis has been obtained. Attention to cardiac function and fluid balance must be meticulous and aggressive. Renal function should return promptly although fluid loading and diuretics are often necessary. Artificial ventilation will be maintained for a period of at least 12–18 hours. There may be a prolonged delay in the resumption of normal gastrointestinal motility but parenteral nutrition is seldom needed. A period of postoperative mental disturbance is common despite adequate oxygenation and the absence of major electrolyte disturbance.

REFERENCES

Collin J 1985 Screening for abdominal aortic aneurysms. British Journal of Surgery 72: 851–852

Crawford E S 1991 Ruptured abdominal aortic aneurysm: an editorial. Journal of Vascular Surgery 13: 348–350

Ingoldby C J H, Wujanto R, Mitchell J E 1986 Impact of vascular surgery on community mortality from ruptured aortic aneurysms. British Journal of Surgery 73: 551–553

Johansen K, Kohler T R, Nicholls S C, Zierler R E, Clowes A W, Kazmers A 1991 Ruptured abdominal aortic aneurysm: the Harborview experience. Journal of Vascular Surgery 13: 240–247

Johnson W C, Gale M E, Gerzof S G, Nabseth D G 1986 The role of computed tomography in symptomatic aortic aneurysms. Surgery, Gynecology and Obstetrics 162: 49–53

Kvilekval K H V, Best I M, Mason R A, Newton G B, Giron F 1990 The value of computed tomography in the management of symptomatic abdominal aortic aneurysms. Journal of Vascular Surgery 12: 28–33

Veith F J, Gupta S K, Wengerter K R 1990 In: Greenhalgh R M, Mannick J A, Powell J T (eds) The cause and management of aneurysms. W B Saunders, London, pp 387–399

PROBLEMS ENCOUNTERED IN ANEURYSM SURGERY

Introduction

Some of the problems encountered during elective and emergency repair of abdominal aortic aneurysm have been described in the previous sections. This section gives an account of several major problems which may be encountered less commonly. These include:

1. Aneurysm close to or involving the renal arteries.
2. Fistula between aorta and major veins.
3. Major venous anomalies and injuries.
4. Horseshoe kidney and renal ectopia.
5. Inflammatory aneurysm.
6. Calcified aorta.
7. Infected aneurysm and aortoenteric fistula.

Chapter 13

Juxtarenal aneurysm

Introduction

In most practices, fewer than 10% of aortic aneurysms involve the renal arteries. On clinical examination, a high aneurysm may be suspected if it is not possible to get the examining fingers between the aneurysm and the costal margin. The role of computed tomographic (CT) scanning, and the problem of the aneurysm which the CT scan falsely indicates to involve the renal arteries, has been described above (see p. 120).

The following discussion is confined to cases where there is a segment of normal or near-normal aorta below the superior mesenteric artery. If this segment is aneurysmal, the patient should be treated as a thoracoabdominal aneurysm (see Ch. 8).

OPERATION

A midline incision is suitable for these patients. The dissection begins as for an elective aneurysm. The left renal vein is mobilized fully as described on page 122. With the left renal vein displaced distally, the aorta above it can be dissected (Fig. 13.1). The ends of the divided inferior mesenteric, left adrenal and left gonadal veins can be seen. The superior mesenteric artery (which lies behind the retractor on the patient's right in Fig. 13.1) is in the base of the small bowel mesentery and limits the amount that the mesentery can be retracted upwards and to the right. The lower border of the pancreas can be mobilized and lifted forwards. The fibres of the crus of the diaphragm to the left of the aorta may be divided. Further dissection around the aorta will allow it to be encircled.

Mobilization of the renal vein as described will provide adequate access in most cases. If it is necessary to divide the renal vein, vascular clamps should be used and the vein rejoined when the aortic anastomoses are complete. There was a time when it was fashionable to divide and ligate the left renal vein. There is no doubt that this manoeuvre improves exposure. However, harmful effects in renal function have been demonstrated although some authors have reported series without demonstrable impairment of renal function.

The proximal parts of each renal artery are dissected. They lie in the mid-lateral plane and can be approached from their inferior surface. Several centimetres of the left renal artery can be displayed after mobilizing the left renal vein (Fig. 13.2a). The proximal part of the right renal artery can be exposed by retracting upwards the junction of the left renal vein and the inferior vena cava (Fig. 13.2b). It is usually possible to display 2–3 cm of the artery from this route. The more extensive exposure provided by approaching the artery from the right side after mobilizing the duodenum and hepatic flexure should not be necessary in these cases.

The preparation of the proximal aorta is complete when the aorta has been controlled, and each renal artery displayed and controlled. Dissection of the distal aorta proceeds as previously described (p. 124).

Aortic anastomosis
Provisional decisions about the types of anastomoses to be performed are made at this stage. The choices include the following:

1. If the aorta is only mildly aneurysmal at the level of the renal arteries, it may be possible to clamp the aorta below the renal arteries and carry out a standard infrarenal repair, fashioning a new neck to the aneurysm with the sutures in the posterior wall. This procedure minimizes the chances of renal ischaemia.
2. The aorta may be clamped above the renal arteries but the anastomosis performed below the renal arteries (Fig. 13.3). This is permissible if the diameter of the aorta at this point will accept a 22 mm graft and if the suture line can be performed safely, without tearing. Sutures must be placed carefully to avoid narrowing the renal artery orifice. Renal ischaemia is reduced to the time taken to perform the proximal anastomosis.

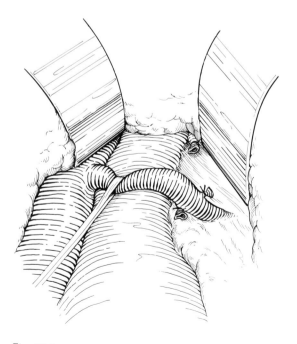

Fig. 13.1
Dissection of suprarenal aorta.

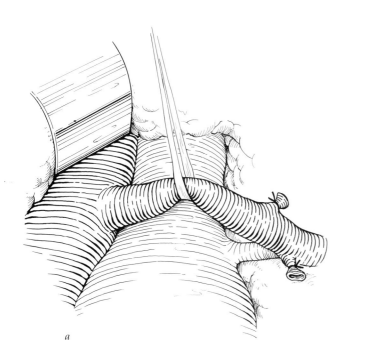

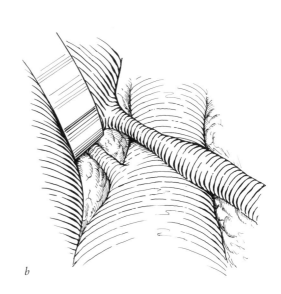

a

b

Fig. 13.2
Dissection of renal arteries. (a) Left. (b) Right.

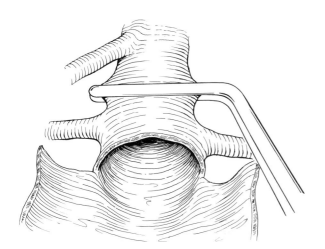

Fig. 13.3
Suprarenal clamp, infrarenal anastomosis.

In many cases it is possible to configure the suture line in such a way that the aneurysmal suprarenal aorta is repaired and the graft fashioned to incorporate both renal arteries above the suture line. Figure 13.4 shows the incision in the anterior wall of the aneurysm. The luminal view before the anastomosis is shown in Figure 13.5. The dotted line indicates the position of the posterior suture line. The insert shows how the graft is fashioned.

3.   It is sometimes possible to clamp the aorta obliquely so that blood flow is maintained to one of the kidneys (usually the right) at all times (Fig. 13.6).

Each of these procedures, if applicable, will lessen the amount of renal ischaemia and this is a highly desirable objective.

4.   If none of these techniques is suitable, the aorta and both renal arteries must be clamped to allow the proximal anastomosis to be performed in optimal conditions. The procedure is now to perform an anastomosis between the proximal aorta and the graft, and to reimplant the renal arteries into the graft. It may be 20–60 minutes between the application of the aortic clamp and the restoration of blood flow to both renal arteries and this carries a risk of renal failure developing.

Preservation of renal function

Several measures to preserve renal function may be undertaken:

1.   The anaesthetist must ensure that the circulating blood volume is adequate to prevent renal vasoconstriction, before application of the clamps.

2.   Mannitol 25% 100 ml may be infused intravenously to ensure the kidneys are in a diuretic phase before they are made ischaemic and to protect from reperfusion injury when blood flow is restored.

3.   Once the aneurysm has been opened, the orifices of the renal arteries may be perfused with 200 ml cold (4°C), lactated, Ringer's solution. This step may be repeated every 20 minutes if necessary. It is not necessary to use solutions developed for prolonged renal preservation. Care should be taken not to damage the renal arteries or to cause embolism.

After the administration of intravenous heparin, clamps are applied to the aorta and renal arteries proximally, and to the iliac arteries distally. The proximal anastomosis to the suprarenal aorta is carried out as described on page 126.

Reimplantation of renal arteries

When the aortic anastomosis is complete (Fig. 13.7) and haemostasis is adequate, the renal arteries are reimplanted. A small circular orifice is cut in the graft at the appropriate level. One of a variety of techniques may be used for the anastomosis:

1.   If the orifice of the renal artery is normal, a Carrel patch may be fashioned as shown in Figure 13.8 and sutured to the graft using monofilament sutures of 4/0 or 5/0. The patch comprises a full-thickness cuff of aortic wall, extending about 3 mm from the orifice of the renal artery. This facilitates placement of the sutures to avoid the orifice of the renal artery.

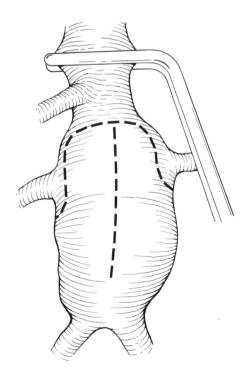

Fig. 13.4
Design of upper anastomosis to include both renal arteries.

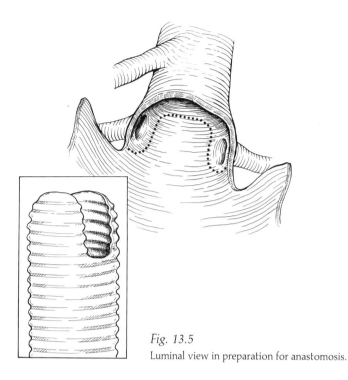

Fig. 13.5
Luminal view in preparation for anastomosis.

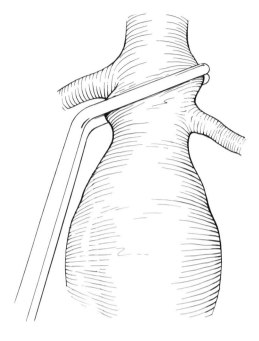

Fig. 13.6
Oblique clamp to aorta.

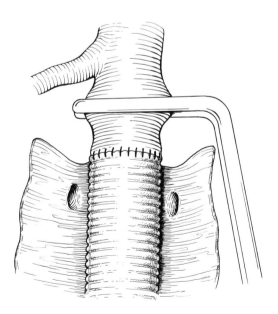

Fig. 13.7
Proximal anastomosis to suprarenal aorta. Renal artery orifices visible.

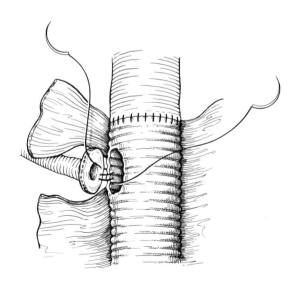

Fig. 13.8
Carrel patch fashioned from wall of aneurysm.

2.   If there is a longer distance from the
anastomosis between aorta and graft to
the site of implantation, it may not be
necessary to divide the aortic wall and
fashion a patch. Instead, the sutures can
be placed through the aortic wall
adjacent to the renal orifice (Fig. 13.9)
(cf. thoracoabdominal aneurysm).

3.   If the orifice of the renal artery is
diseased and stenosed, the artery may
be transected through an area relatively
free of disease, and the cut end sutured
to the graft. Occasionally the artery is
too short and a small interposition graft
of saphenous vein should be used.
Alternatively, an endarterectomy by
eversion of the orifice may be
performed.

Care must be taken to prevent
embolism of the renal arteries. Careful
removal of loose debris, back-bleeding
and gentle flushing of the renal arteries
should be undertaken.

After the first anastomosis has been
completed, blood flow should be
restored to the kidney by oblique
placement of the aortic clamp as shown
in Figure 13.10.

When both renal anastomoses are
complete, the graft should be clamped
below them and the lower anastomosis
carried out as described on page 128.

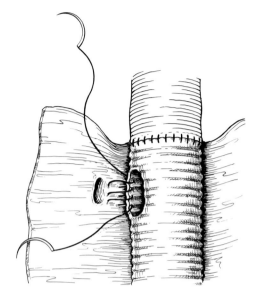

Fig. 13.9
Suturing around orifice of renal artery.

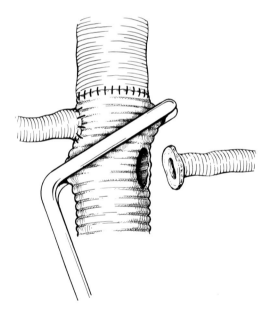

Fig. 13.10
Restoration of flow to the right renal artery.

Chapter 14

Aortocaval fistula

Introduction

In about 1% of patients with abdominal aortic aneurysm, a connection between the aneurysm and a major vein may occur. One of three sites may be involved:

1.   Aorta to inferior vena cava or common iliac vein.
2.   Common iliac artery to common iliac vein.
3.   Aorta to left renal vein (Merrill & Ernst 1981).

An aortocaval fistula is the commonest of these conditions. Fistula may also occur as the result of trauma either from gunshot wounds or, more commonly, following surgery on a lumbar disc.

PATHOLOGY

The pathology can be considered as erosion of the aneurysm into the inferior vena cava. When the thrombus has been removed from an abdominal aortic aneurysm, it is common to find the anterior longitudinal ligament of the spinal column in the base of the wound. In the same way, the wall between the aorta and the inferior vena cava may be eroded but occluded by thrombus in the lumen of the aneurysm.

In cases of traumatic origin, the missile or surgical instrument perforates both aorta and inferior vena cava or common iliac vein. Fistula following surgery occurs in the region of the aortic bifurcation but lesions from gunshot wounds may occur at any point along the aorta.

CLINICAL FEATURES

The clinical picture may be quite variable, although the haemodynamic effects of the shunts have been well characterized. Aortocaval fistulae tend to present acutely but iliac fistulae may be present for months before diagnosis. Back pain is the predominant clinical feature. The pain may radiate to the loin or down the leg. The most characteristic finding is a harsh abdominal bruit which may be heard in 80% of cases. The aortic aneurysm tends to be large and therefore easily palpable on abdominal examination. High-output heart failure is present in about one-third of cases. Oedema and cyanosis of the lower limbs will be present in about 40% and pulsating varicose veins (unilateral if the fistula is to a common iliac vein) may be seen. Haematuria and renal failure each occur in about one-third of cases. Pulmonary embolism from expulsion of thrombus from within the aneurysm to the vena cava is a rare but well-documented event. Closure of the fistula results in prompt reversal of the haemodynamic effects.

Only very few patients have been reported with a fistula between the aorta and the left renal vein. The characteristic symptoms suggest pain arising from the kidney or ureter. The possibility of a renal origin for the symptoms is increased by the finding of microscopic haematuria.

The acute presentation may have features of a ruptured aneurysm, with back pain and collapse with hypotension. At operation there are no signs of rupture of the aneurysm to the retroperitoneal tissues. The key finding is the palpation of a thrill in the inferior vena cava. This enables a confident diagnosis to be made.

The condition may not be diagnosed until, during an elective operation to repair an abdominal aortic aneurysm,

removal of the intraluminal thrombus is followed by profuse venous haemorrhage. In these cases the opening between aorta and inferior vena cava has been occluded by the thrombus, so that the fistula did not exist before the thrombus was removed.

INVESTIGATIONS

If an aortogram is performed, the early filling of the inferior vena cava will indicate the presence of a fistula. Proteinuria may result from the increased pressure in the renal veins.

PREOPERATIVE PREPARATION

If the diagnosis is made preoperatively, a Swan–Ganz catheter should be inserted to enable precise monitoring of cardiac function and to guide fluid replacement (see p. 19). The characteristic finding is a high cardiac output and a low peripheral resistance. Preoperative monitoring will allow cardiac function to be improved and the optimal time for surgery chosen.

OPERATION

The dissection of the aorta and iliac vessels proceeds as described on page 122. This may be more difficult than usual because of the venous hypertension which causes bleeding from small veins. The important step is to minimize venous haemorrhage while the fistula is closed: substantial blood loss has been reported in most of these procedures. There are several ways in which this may be done:

1.   The safest way is to dissect and isolate the vena cava. Dissection of the inferior vena cava above the fistula and below the renal veins is straightforward. The adventitial tissues are divided and the inferior vena cava mobilized

(Fig. 14.1). The major danger is tearing of lumbar veins, one of which can be seen in the figure. This can be prevented if the dissection is very gentle and there are no attempts to pass instruments blindly around the inferior vena cava. It may be possible to place a tape around the inferior vena cava, although sufficient dissection to allow the safe application of a clamp is appropriate. It should be emphasized that no attempt should be made to dissect directly the venous side of the fistula.

The vessels below the fistula are dissected sufficiently to allow *adequate* digital compression by fingers placed on either side of the right common iliac artery in the sites indicated in

Figure 14.2. Formal dissection and control of both common iliac veins is hazardous, and adequate compression can be achieved against the vertebral column, provided the position of the veins is identified.

If the aneurysm is opened before the fistula is discovered, the wall of the aneurysm should be closed with large clamps as shown in Figure 14.1. This will control venous bleeding while the dissection is performed.

2.   The fistula may be controlled by passing balloon catheters proximally and distally into the inferior vena cava after opening the aorta (Fig. 14.2). This technique has been reported to work satisfactorily. It may be difficult to

maintain the position of the catheters, as these are manoeuvres which are not practised frequently. For these reasons, it is probably safer to use the technique described above.

The most rapid method of closing the fistula is for the surgeon to place a finger in the defect and insert the sutures while the fistula is being occluded in this way. This may not be satisfactory, because it may be very difficult to place the sutures accurately while occluding the fistula, and the net result may be greater blood loss. It may be applicable to very small (1 cm or less) fistulae.

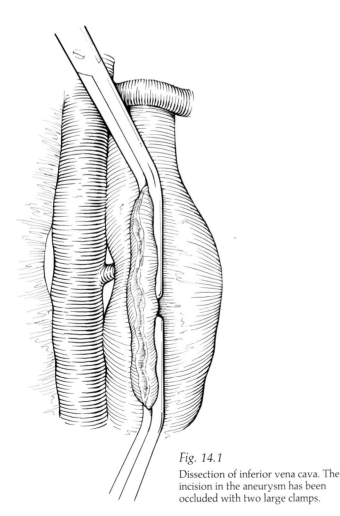

Fig. 14.1
Dissection of inferior vena cava. The incision in the aneurysm has been occluded with two large clamps.

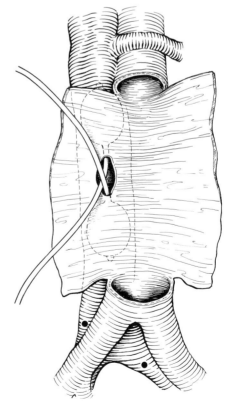

Fig. 14.2
Anatomy of aortocaval fistula in right posterolateral aspect of aneurysm. Foley balloon catheters have been inserted to control bleeding.

The fistula is usually 2 cm or more long and at least 1 cm wide. The margins comprise the wall of both the aneurysm and the inferior vena cava. Because of the size of the defect to be closed, it is important to take thick bites of the aortic wall to ensure a secure closure: bites that are too fine will tear out. Three or four sutures are usually required. They may be tied as they are placed (Fig. 14.3a) or the ends may be held long and all the sutures tied after they have all been placed (Fig. 14.3b).

Compression of the iliac veins can be relaxed (much to the relief of the assistant who has been performing that task) and the caval clamp removed. The operation then proceeds as for an elective repair.

A fistula involving a common iliac vein is dealt with in a similar manner.

In fistula due to trauma the principles of the repair are similar. However, it is not always possible to repair the veins and venous ligation is necessary in about one-third of patients (Brewster et al 1991). The damaged arterial segment may also need to be replaced by a short bypass graft.

A fistula to the left renal vein is usually to a retroaortic left renal vein (see p. 172). Closure of the fistula from within the aneurysm is usually straightforward. The aortic clamp may need to be placed above the renal arteries. Dissection of the renal vein is not advocated because of the difficulties of this procedure and the ease of control of the fistula once the aneurysm has been opened.

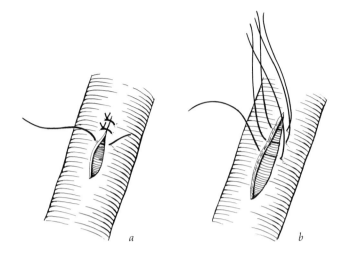

Fig. 14.3
Closure of fistula. (a) Interrupted sutures tied as they are placed. (b) Sutures all placed before they are tied.

REFERENCES

Brewster D C, Cambria R P, Moncure A C et al 1991 Aortocaval and iliac arteriovenous fistulas: recognition and treatment. Journal of Vascular Surgery 13: 253–265
Merrill W H, Ernst C B 1981 Aorta–left renal vein fistula: hemodynamic monitoring and timing of operation. Surgery 89: 678–682

Chapter 15

Major vein anomalies and injuries

Introduction

Major venous bleeding is a serious complication of vascular surgery. It may be more difficult to control than arterial bleeding and usually results in substantial blood loss. It may be considered under two headings:

1.　Bleeding from veins in their normal anatomical position.
2.　Bleeding from abnormal veins.

The incidence of major venous tears in the region of the inferior vena cava has been reduced by the adoption of intraluminal techniques for the replacement of abdominal aortic aneurysm. Tears in the region of the iliac veins still occur during dissection of these structures. Major venous bleeding from the region of the neck of the aneurysm may be coming from congenital abnormalities of the veins in this region, as well as from normally positioned veins. Damage to abnormal veins occurs characteristically before the anomaly is recognized. The presence of these anomalies is one of the reasons why the technique of minimal dissection of the region of the neck of an aneurysm has been advocated.

EMBRYOLOGY

The understanding of the anomalies encountered depends on knowledge of the embryology of the veins in the region (Chuang et al 1974).

1.   The earliest veins are the paired posterior cardinal veins (A), which drain the caudal part of the embryo, receiving tributaries from the lower limb bud, pelvis and mesonephros. They run in the dorsal part of the mesonephric ridge and appear in a 4 mm embryo (4–5 weeks' gestation). The anastomosis between the posterior cardinal veins persists in the adult as the left common iliac vein. The cranial ends of the vein persist on the left as the superior intercostal vein, and on the right as the proximal part of the azygos vein. The cranial end of the ureter lies dorsal to the posterior cardinal veins, but distally the ureter passes in front of the veins (Fig. 15.1a).

2.   A second pair of veins, the subcardinal veins (B), lie ventrally and medially in the mesonephric ridge, and communicate with the posterior cardinal veins and with each other in front of the aorta. These veins become larger and take over the drainage of the mesonephros as the posterior cardinal veins regress. The anastomosis in front of the aorta persists as the left renal vein. The adrenal veins cranially and the gonadal veins caudally join the subcardinal veins.

3.   The proximal part of the right subcardinal system comes into relationship with the liver and its veins. In this way the right-sided veins present a more direct pathway to the heart and enlarge, while the veins on the left side tend to regress.

4.   The supracardinal veins (C) appear lateral to the aorta and the sympathetic trunks. They communicate caudally with the iliac veins and cranially with the posterior cardinal veins. Communications occur with the subcardinal veins in the region of the preaortic inter-subcardinal anastomosis. This anastomosis, together with the inter-supracardinal anastomoses behind the aorta, forms the 'renal collar'. The caudal part of the left supracardinal vein regresses.

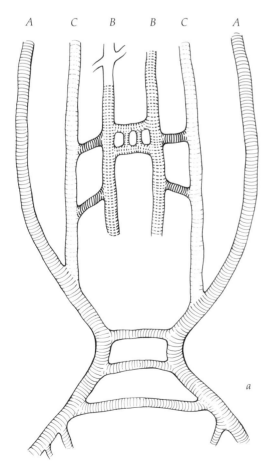

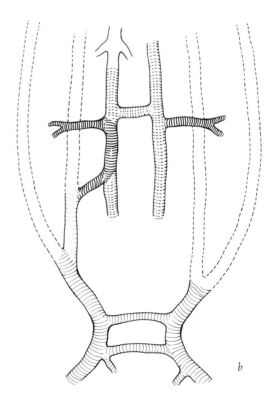

Fig. 15.1
Embryology of the inferior vena cava.

5.   The anastomoses between the supracardinal and subcardinal veins form the area of the renal veins and, on the right side, part of the inferior vena cava. Caudal to this segment the right supracardinal vein forms the inferior vena cava (Fig. 15.1b).

The common iliac veins and inferior vena cava are developed in their adult pattern (Fig. 15.2) in an 18–20 mm embryo (Bartle et al 1987) and are derived from:

a.   The posterior cardinal veins and the anastomosis between them (A).
b.   The right supracardinal vein (C).
c.   The anastomoses between the right supracardinal and subcardinal veins.
d.   The right subcardinal vein (B) which receives the left renal vein derived from the inter-subcardinal anastomosis.
e.   The hepatic veins.

The renal collar is derived from:

a.   The subcardinal–supracardinal anastomoses forming the inferior vena cava on the right and part of the left renal vein on the left.
b.   Anteriorly, the inter-subcardinal anastomoses forming the left renal vein.
c.   Posteriorly, the inter-supracardinal anastomoses persisting as the central parts of the left lumbar veins.
d.   On the left side the tributary connecting the left renal vein and the lumbar or azygos system (see Fig. 9.3).

ANOMALIES

With the complicated development of the inferior vena cava, many abnormalities are possible. However, only a few are of clinical importance.

Anomalies of the infrarenal inferior vena cava
Persisting right posterior cardinal vein
This anomaly results from persistence of the posterior cardinal vein forming the

inferior vena cava in the segment normally formed by the supracardinal vein. The posterior cardinal vein joins the area of the anastomosis between the subcardinal and supracardinal veins. As a consequence, the right ureter runs behind the inferior vena cava and descends medial to it, resulting in the anomaly called 'retrocaval ureter'.

Persisting left supracardinal vein
This results in a *left-sided inferior vena cava* which receives the left renal vein and crosses the aorta to meet a normal suprarenal inferior vena cava (Fig. 15.3). It may cross either in front of or behind the aorta (Brener et al 1974).

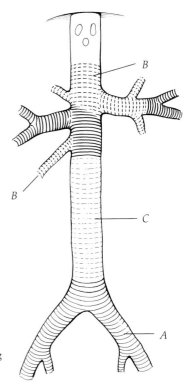

Fig. 15.2
Inferior vena cava showing embryonic origin of various parts.

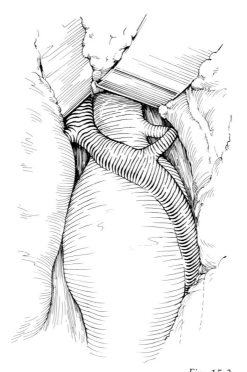

Fig. 15.3
Left-sided inferior vena cava.

Persisting right and left supracardinal veins
This results in a *double inferior vena cava*. The left-sided division joins the left renal vein as in a left-sided inferior vena cava. This is the commonest of this group of abnormalities, its incidence being estimated at 1–3% (Chuang et al 1974). There may be one or more communications in front of the aorta between the two divisions.

Abnormalities of anastomosis between posterior cardinal veins
The network of veins in the region of the bifurcation of the aorta may persist as a left common iliac vein which passes anterior to the right common iliac artery. In some cases there may be veins both anterior and posterior to the artery.

Anomalies of the renal collar
The normal anatomy results from regression of the posterior component of the renal collar and development of the anterior component. Anomalies may result from:

1. Regression of the anterior component giving a *retroaortic left renal vein*. The incidence of this is about 2%.
2. Persistence of both components giving a *circumaortic venous ring*. When large, this vein commonly runs caudally to join the lower part of the inferior vena cava (Brener et al 1974). It is usually joined by large lumbar and retroperitoneal veins. The left subcardinal–supracardinal anastomosis often persists as a small branch from the left side of the left renal vein to a lumbar vein. This represents a rudimentary circumaortic venous ring and is the commonest of the anomalies of the renal collar. It is said to occur in up to 16% of subjects but anecdotal experience of the retroperitoneal approach to the aorta, when it is a useful guide to the position of the left renal artery (Fig. 9.3), suggests that it is more common. Its importance is that it limits the mobility of the left renal vein and may cause

troublesome bleeding if torn. Its approximate position is indicated in Figure 10.4 and its presence should always be remembered when the left renal vein is being mobilized.

Abnormalities of suprarenal inferior vena cava
If there is failure of the anastomosis between the right subcardinal vein and the hepatic vein, this segment of the inferior vena cava does not develop. Proximal venous drainage is through the cranial portions of the supracardinal veins which develop into the azygos and hemiazygos veins.

SURGICAL SIGNIFICANCE

The first sign of the presence of one of these anomalies may be the presence of venous haemorrhage, as a result of injuring a major vein.

DIAGNOSIS

It is rare for any of these anomalies to be diagnosed preoperatively. However, the major anomalies may be seen on computed tomographic (CT) scans (Bartle et al 1987). When dissecting the neck of an aneurysm, the possibility of venous anomalies should be remembered. Any hint of abnormality, such as a small left renal vein or large veins to the left aorta, should result in a planned dissection to carefully delineate the anatomy.

PREVENTION OF INJURY

The common sites of injury are shown in Figure 15.4. Because of the seriousness of these tears, techniques of dissection which minimize the chances of them happening should be adopted. The technique of minimal dissection of the iliac arteries (p. 124) is one such step. Dissection of the distal common iliac artery is often easier because the vein and artery are less adherent, and venous bleeding is easier to control further from the bifurcation. The other steps include strict observance of the fundamental rules of dissection in vascular surgery, namely keeping the dissection as close as possible to the wall of the artery and never attempting to pass an instrument blindly around an artery. Adherence to these principles should minimize injuries to veins.

Renal collar
The small retroaortic branch of the left renal vein can be found just to the left of the aorta. Mobilization of the left renal vein in this area should be carried out carefully and, if the vein is identified, it should be dissected, ligated and divided.

An absent (anterior) left renal vein should not interfere with the conduct of the operation. Care should be taken if the aorta is to be encircled, but, as described above, the retroaortic left renal vein commonly runs caudally, and therefore away from the area of the dissection, thus improving access to the renal arteries. However, injury to this vein may be very difficult to control. The best solution may be to transect the aorta and directly expose the area of injury.

Double or left-sided inferior vena cava
A left-sided inferior vena cava (Fig. 15.3) commonly crosses the aorta at the level of the neck of an aneurysm. It may be possible to mobilize the vessel sufficiently to allow adequate access to

the aorta. Access may be improved by dividing the right renal vein. If the exposure is not satisfactory, it may be necessary to divide the inferior vena cava. Complete ligation of the inferior vena cava will result in venous hypertension, and ulceration in the lower limbs will occur in about one-third of the cases.

If there is a double inferior vena cava, the left component may be divided. This should not produce any serious consequences, provided that the left pelvic venous system anastomoses with the right.

MANAGEMENT

The management of tears when they occur may be very difficult. The first step is to apply pressure to the area with packs, advise the anaesthetist of the likelihood of substantial blood loss and ensure that two functioning suction systems are available. Once the anaesthetist has made any necessary adjustments, the packs are removed and the area inspected. An attempt is made to confine the bleeding by proximal and distal compression of the vein digitally, or by means of swabs attached to sponge-holding forceps. The site of the bleeding is inspected and appropriate dissection is performed to allow optimal visibility of the area.

In many cases the cause is avulsion of a tributary (Fig. 15.5a, b). The best solution is to grasp the vein with a curved vascular clamp so that the site of the hole is within the clamp (Fig. 15.5c, d). It does not matter if the vein is partly or totally occluded by the clamp. As a consequence of applying the clamp, the bleeding is controlled and the defect can be sutured under optimal conditions (Fig. 15.5e).

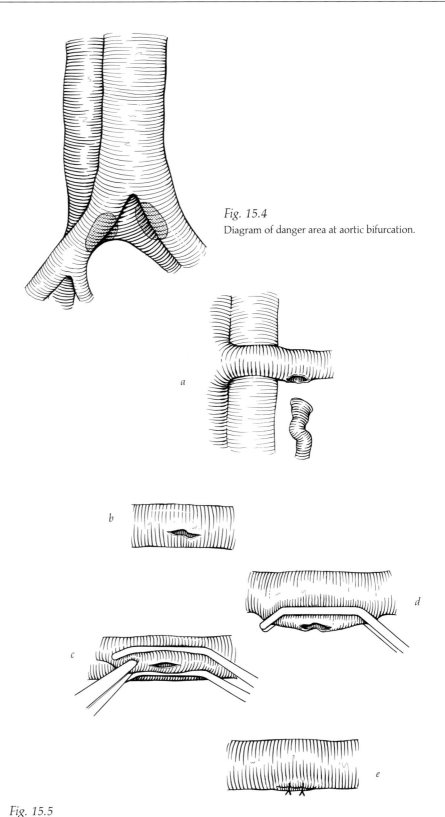

Fig. 15.4
Diagram of danger area at aortic bifurcation.

Fig. 15.5
Avulsion of gonadal vein and repair. (a) Diagram illustrating site of avulsion. (b) Identification of hole. (c) Application of clamp. (d) Clamp applied to control bleeding and display hole. (e) Vein repaired, clamp removed.

Control is not usually so easy in the area beneath the aortic bifurcation because it may be impossible to apply safely an effective clamp. In this situation, it may be necessary to control the inferior vena cava and both common iliac veins, in order to produce sufficient mobilization to apply a clamp across the defect. While the area of the tear is compressed by means of swabs attached to sponge-holding forceps, the veins are dissected. This should be carried out sufficiently to allow the veins to be compressed or clamped as described on page 165. This may produce sufficient mobility to allow a clamp to be applied across the damaged area as described above. Sometimes the repair must be performed with the vessels digitally compressed. To obtain access to the confluence of the common iliac veins, it may be necessary to divide the right common iliac artery and dissect it forwards away from the veins (Fig. 15.6).

Placement of the sutures may be difficult. Suturing deep in the wound, with restricted access and less than perfect haemostasis, presents a considerable challenge. To add to the difficulties, the veins are thin walled and fragile, so that they are very easily torn by the needle or in the act of tying the suture. Sometimes the problems of achieving haemostasis result in a deliberate decision to ligate the vein(s) and accept the probable consequences from venous insufficiency in the lower limb(s).

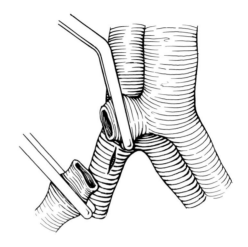

Fig. 15.6
Division of right common iliac artery to allow access to tear.

REFERENCES

Bartle E J, Pearce W H, Sun J H, Rutherford R B 1987 Journal of Vascular Surgery 6: 590–593
Brener B J, Darling R C, Frederick P L, Linton R R 1974 Major venous abnormalities complicating abdominal aortic surgery. Archives of Surgery 108: 159–165
Chuang V P, Mena C E, Hoskins P A 1974 Congenital anomalies of the inferior vena cava: review of embryogenesis and presentation of a simplified classification. British Journal of Radiology 47: 206–213

Chapter 16

Horseshoe kidney and renal ectopia

1. HORSESHOE KIDNEY

This is the commonest of the anomalies of renal ascent and fusion and has been reported in 1:700 unselected autopsies. The elements of the lesion are fusion of varying extent, renal masses on each side of the vertebral column and ureters which do not cross the midline. Embryologically it results from partial fusion of the nephrogenic elements before they migrate cranially. The primitive segmental blood supply to the kidneys may persist in part, so that there may be multiple renal arteries and veins.

In an operation on the aorta, the presence of any of these anomalies may complicate the surgery, because the presence of renal tissue and its associated vessels and ureters hinders direct access to the anterior aspect of the aorta. In early reports of the combination of aortic disease and horseshoe kidney, substantial numbers of patients were considered inoperable, or division of the isthmus was considered necessary. Modern techniques should allow operation to be performed without division of the renal isthmus.

DIAGNOSIS

The diagnosis is readily made on computed tomographic (CT) scan by the presence of renal tissue, anterior to the aorta. The renal tissue is identified by being contiguous with the kidney(s) and with an image that is enhanced following intravenous injection of contrast. If pyelography is performed, the classic sign is the presence of one or more calyces medial to the ureter.

If these conditions are suspected, angiography is mandatory to delineate the blood supply to the renal tissue because these vessels must be preserved during resection of the aneurysm.

ANATOMY

Arteries
This information comes from the series on horseshoe kidney reported by Eisendrath et al (1925) and Connelly et al (1980). The renal vessels may arise in the normal position, from the lower aorta laterally or anteriorly and from the iliac arteries. The common patterns are:

1.   Normal renal artery on each side (20%) (Fig. 16.1a).
2.   Normal renal artery on each side plus a single artery to the isthmus arising from the aorta (30%).
3.   Two arteries from the aorta to each side of the kidney plus a single artery to the isthmus arising from the aorta (15%) (Fig. 16.1b).
4.   Two renal arteries arising from the aorta and/or iliac arteries and one or two to the isthmus arising from the iliac arteries (15%).
5.   Six to eight arteries arising from both aorta and iliac arteries (20%).

Summarizing this information:

1.   A single normal renal artery to each side is present in 50–75% of cases (Connelly et al 1980).
2.   The isthmus will not have a separate blood supply, or will be supplied by a single vessel arising from the aorta in 65% of cases.

Veins
The anatomy of the veins in these patients is not well described, yet at operation the veins are much more prominent than the arteries (Fig. 16.2). The left renal vein usually runs from low on the left side of the aorta, to the inferior vena cava in the normal position. It runs across the anterior aspect of the aneurysm. The veins from the right side run upwards, lateral to the aorta, to join the inferior vena cava. The veins from the isthmus drain upwards, to the left renal vein or the inferior vena cava. There are usually a number of large veins in the area between the renal tissue. These may also drain posteriorly via a variable number of tributaries to the lumbar plexus.

Ureters
The renal pelvis lies anteriorly in the renal hilum. The ureters usually pass anterior to the isthmus and cross the common iliac arteries in the normal region (Fig. 16.2). Multiple ectopic ureters are rare.

OPERATION

The initial stages of the operation, including the mobilization of the duodenum, are carried out in the routine manner. The masses of renal tissue will be seen anterior to the aorta. Fatty tissue containing arteries, veins and urinary drainage systems will be present in the region between the two renal masses.

The aorta is dissected above the neck of the aneurysm. As this is being carried out, a careful search should be made along the sides of the aorta for renal arteries which may be close to the aorta as they run obliquely downwards. The left renal vein may or may not be in its normal position. A tape is passed around the aorta.

The dissection should identify all the significant renal arteries. The findings of the preoperative angiography will assist this process but it is wise not to assume that the arteriogram has identified all the important arteries (Crawford et al 1988). The area between the renal masses is dissected. The adipose tissue is dissected away from the veins, which are the most prominent structures encountered. The aim of the dissection

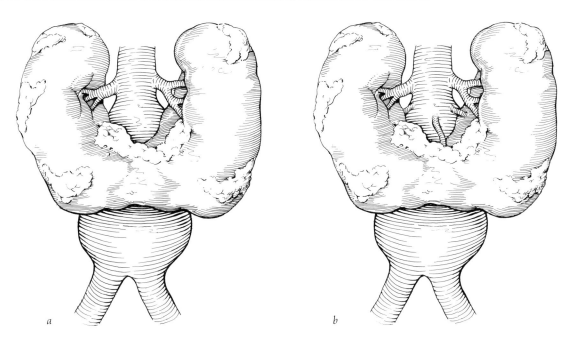

Fig. 16.1
Arterial anatomy. (a) Single renal artery on each side. (b) Two renal arteries on each side, one to isthmus. Lower arteries and artery to isthmus will need to be reimplanted.

is to dissect away the adipose tissue and mobilize the veins, in order to expose the anterior aspect of the aorta and identify arteries arising from it.

The isthmus is mobilized from the aorta. There is a plane of loose areolar tissue between the renal tissue and the aorta. This loose tissue is divided inferior to the isthmus and the renal mass lifted forwards. Dissection is carried out both above and below the isthmus. Care is taken to identify any renal arteries which may be found during dissection. The ureters should be identified anterior to the isthmus. In about one-third of the reported cases (Connelly et al 1980) the isthmus was resected, apparently without serious sequelae. In some cases, the isthmus is thin and fibrous and this can be divided easily. If the isthmus contains substantial amounts of renal parenchyma it should be preserved. Irreparable damage to a significant renal artery may require resection of the ischaemic segment.

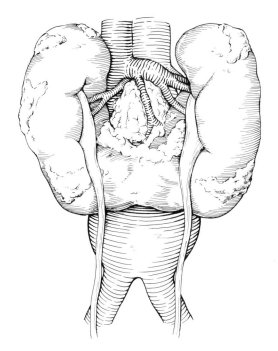

Fig. 16.2
Anatomy of veins and ureters. Anterior aspect of aneurysm is covered by veins, ureters and adipose tissue in addition to isthmus.

The iliac vessels are dissected in the usual manner.

Once this dissection has been completed, the surgeon should pause to plan how best to preserve the renal arteries:

1. The principal renal arteries will be left in place above the graft.
2. The vessel(s) arising from the front or side of the aorta can either be incorporated in the proximal suture line or preserved on a Carrel patch (see p. 159) and anastomosed to a hole cut in the anterior aspect of the graft.
3. If there are significant renal vessels arising from the iliac arteries, they will be preserved if the lower anastomosis is to the aortic bifurcation.
4. Multiple small vessels running to the isthmus may be divided.

Clamps are applied to the aorta and iliac arteries in the usual way. Clamps are also applied to renal arteries which arise from the aorta in the isolated segment. The isthmus is lifted forwards and the anterior wall of the aneurysm is incised. Lumbar arteries are oversewn. Other sites of significant back-bleeding should be examined carefully, to ensure that they do not represent the orifice(s) of accessory renal arteries which have not been identified previously. Such vessels should be preserved.

The proximal anastomosis is performed. This can usually be carried out from the anterior approach. The graft may be placed in the lumen of the aneurysm, deep to the isthmus, or, if space allows, the graft may remain superficial to the isthmus and be moved as described on page 126 during the performance of the anastomosis.

If there is insufficient access to the neck of the aneurysm from the anterior approach, the aorta should be approached in the retroperitoneal plane, after mobilizing the left colon and spleen. The left renal mass is mobilized forwards and this will provide good access to the neck of the aneurysm. The retroperitoneal exposure should not be used for the initial approach because of the difficulty in identifying the renal arteries, especially on the right side.

Following completion of the proximal anastomosis, the graft should be placed deep to the isthmus and reimplantation of arteries performed if necessary (Fig. 16.3).

The proximal clamp is removed and the graft clamped distal to the reimplanted renal arteries. The distal anastomosis proceeds in the usual manner. The wall of the aneurysm should be used to cover the anastomoses.

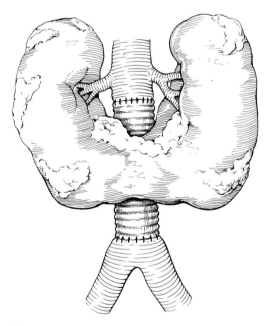

Fig. 16.3
Completed graft lying behind isthmus.

2. RENAL ECTOPIA

PELVIC KIDNEY (INCLUDING RENAL TRANSPLANT)

The incidence of pelvic kidney is between 1:2000 and 1:3000. Occasional cases have been reported associated with aortic aneurysm. The commonest cause of pelvic kidney at the present time is a renal transplant. The surgical approach is similar to that described above. It is essential to identify and preserve the arteries to the kidney.

Renal perfusion may be preserved during performance of the proximal anastomosis by the 'double clamping' technique described by LaCombe (1985). Two clamps (or a clamp and a staple line) are applied to the neck of the aneurysm (Fig. 16.4). Note that the neck of the aneurysm is transected to allow adequate access for the proximal anastomosis. The kidney is perfused via lumbar and inferior mesenteric arteries and collaterals entering the iliac arteries. Cold perfusion of the renal artery may also be used.

The renal arteries are reattached using one of the techniques described on page 158.

CROSSED RENAL ECTOPIA

This heading, which implies that one of the renal masses is on the opposite side of the body to that on which it developed in intrauterine life, includes a wide variety of anomalies. The renal masses may be anywhere between the pelvis and the diaphragm, they may represent one or both kidneys, and they may or may not be fused together. Because they represent abnormalities of migration, there may also be a wide variation in the blood supply and the ureteric drainage.

The blood supply to the kidneys is unpredictable and usually anomalous. Thus the principles described for the other renal abnormalities apply to this condition.

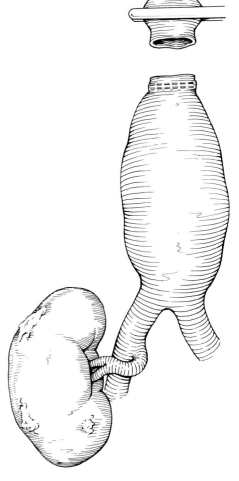

Fig. 16.4
Double-clamping of aorta to permit perfusion of distally placed renal artery.

REFERENCES

Connelly T L, McKinnon W, Smith R B, Perdue G D 1980 Abdominal aortic surgery and horseshoe kidney: a report of six cases and a review. Archives of Surgery 115: 1459–1463
Crawford E S, Coselli J S, Safi H J, Martin T D, Pool J L 1988 The impact of renal fusion and ectopia on aortic surgery. Journal of Vascular Surgery 8: 375–383
Eisendrath D N, Phifer F M, Culver H B 1925 Horseshoe kidney. Annals of Surgery 82: 735–764
LaCombe M 1985 Abdominal aortic aneurysmectomy in renal transplant patients. Annals of Surgery 203: 62–68

Chapter 17

Inflammatory aneurysm

Introduction

About 5% of abdominal aortic aneurysms will have a thick fibrotic component in the wall. These are called inflammatory aneurysms (syn. perianeurysmal fibrosis, chronic periaortitis) (see Pennell et al 1985 and Lindblad et al 1991 for review). The extent of the fibrosis may vary, from a plaque several centimetres in diameter on the wall of the aneurysm, to an extensive pannus of tissue. In addition to the aorta, this may involve the duodenum (80–90%), the left renal vein (40–50%), the inferior vena cava (33–60%) and one ureter (20%) or both ureters (a further 20%). Histologically, the pannus comprises thick collagenous tissue with a chronic inflammatory reaction, including lymphocytes and plasma cells. These findings are identical to the features of the condition of idiopathic retroperitoneal fibrosis. The aetiology of the lesion is unknown. Hypotheses which have been proposed include an autoimmune reaction to lipid in the arterial wall, response to repeated intramural haemorrhage and lymphatic stasis.

CLINICAL FEATURES

There are no specific features in the clinical picture which are diagnostic of inflammatory aneurysm. They are more commonly symptomatic than non-inflammatory aneurysms. Back pain is a prominent symptom (76%) and may be accompanied by high erythrocyte sedimentation rate (26%). The serum creatinine is raised in about 30% and occasionally the patient presents with renal failure due to bilateral ureteric obstruction. In most cases, the diagnosis is made on the basis of the preoperative computed tomographic (CT) scan or at operation.

INVESTIGATIONS

CT scanning will show the thick pannus of connective tissue located in the anterior and lateral walls of the aneurysm. The tissue has a high radiological density during contrast infusion. This finding is highly specific but the examination is not very sensitive (20–50%), although Baskerville et al (1983) reported no false-negative examinations in 15 cases. Ultrasound examination may occasionally demonstrate the thick aortic wall or, more frequently, the presence of ureteric obstruction.

TREATMENT

Steroid therapy may produce rapid remission of symptoms and reduce the amount of fibrosis, thus facilitating an operation performed at a later date (Baskerville et al 1983).

The natural history of these aneurysms is uncertain but there is evidence that they are less likely to rupture than ordinary aneurysms. Following repair, the long-term survival is similar in both inflammatory and non-inflammatory aneurysms (Pennell et al 1985).

OPERATION

The lack of specificity in the clinical features and investigations means that a correct preoperative diagnosis is made in only about 30% of cases. Thus any surgeon undertaking repair of an abdominal aortic aneurysm must be prepared to deal with this complication. Small areas of fibrous pannus may be ignored and the operation proceed in a routine manner. Operation in these patients takes longer, and more blood is lost, than in a non-inflammatory abdominal aortic aneurysm.

Technical difficulties arise if the fibrosis is so extensive that it incorporates the duodenum and involves the region of the neck of the aneurysm. This occurs in about half the patients with duodenal involvement. In these cases, the standard advice is that no attempt to free the duodenum should be made. The sides of the aorta are less involved in the inflammatory process. Dissection in the tissues to the left of the aorta will usually allow the infrarenal aorta to be dissected (Fig. 17.1). In many cases, a window can be dissected to allow the safe application of a clamp above the duodenum in the region of the junction of the left renal vein and the inferior vena cava. In the more extensive cases, suprarenal or supracoeliac clamping (see p. 144) should be employed.

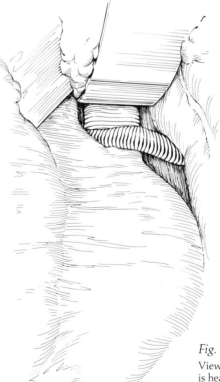

Fig. 17.1
View of inflammatory pannus. The duodenum is heavily involved but there is an area free of fibrosis between the left renal vein and the aneurysm.

Sometimes it is possible to safely dissect the duodenum from the aneurysm. If this is possible it should be carried out. The plane of the dissection is through the fibrous tissue in the aortic wall, well away from the wall of the duodenum. A hole in the duodenum is potentially catastrophic and is to be avoided.

If the diagnosis is made preoperatively, and if there are indications that the duodenum is involved, a retroperitoneal approach (see p. 109) may be used. This approach is facilitated by the observation that the sides of the aneurysm are less involved in the inflammatory process.

It is usually possible to carry out the distal anastomosis in the routine manner, although difficulty as a consequence of involvement of the distal vessels has been described in about one-third of cases. In these circumstances, dissection in the region of the distal common iliac artery should not be undertaken lest the ureters be damaged. The external iliac arteries should be dissected and clamped. If there is back-bleeding from the internal iliac arteries, this can be controlled by the insertion of balloon catheters into the orifice of the common iliac arteries.

The place of ureterolysis is controversial. Lindblad et al (1991) found that ureterolysis did not affect the postoperative serum creatinine levels. It is stated that the fibrosis will regress following resection of the aneurysm. This suggests that routine ureterolysis is not necessary. It may be necessary to place ureteric catheters preoperatively, to ensure unobstructed flow of urine during the perioperative period. If ureterolysis is carried out, the dissection should not be too close to the wall of the ureter, for fear of damaging either the ureter or its blood supply.

RESULTS

The mortality following surgery is higher than for non-inflammatory aneurysms, presumably as a consequence of technical difficulties encountered during the operation (Fiorani et al 1990, Lindblad et al 1991).

REFERENCES

Baskerville P A, Blakeney C G, Young A E, Browse N L 1983 The diagnosis and treatment of periaortic fibrosis ('inflammatory' aneurysms). British Journal of Surgery 70: 381–385

Fiorani P, Lauri D, Faraglia V, De Santis F, Massucci M, Speziale F 1990 In: Greenhalgh R M, Mannick J A, Powell J T (eds) The cause and management of aneurysms. W B Saunders, London, pp 189–202

Lindblad B, Almgren B, Bergqvist D et al 1991 Abdominal aortic aneurysm with periaortic fibrosis: experience from 11 Swedish vascular centres. Journal of Vascular Surgery 13: 231–239

Pannell R C, Hollier L H, Lie J T et al 1985 Inflammatory abdominal aortic aneurysms: a thirty-year review. Journal of Vascular Surgery 2: 859–869

Chapter 18

Calcified aorta

Introduction

Calcification is a common feature of the pathology of atherosclerosis. The diagnosis of abdominal aortic aneurysm on plain film of the abdomen depends on the presence of this form of calcification. The common pattern seen is the calcification in the atheromatous plaques, which appears as irregular lumps of calcification. This is in contrast to the calcification of the tunica media, a characteristic feature of vascular calcification in diabetes mellitus, which appears on radiographs as fine speckled calcification of arteries of the lower limb.

OPERATION

Calcification may cause serious technical problems in the performance of an anastomosis, although this is much more common in the performance of a side-to-end bypass from the aorta to an aortofemoral bypass graft. The problem is noted when the needle cannot be passed through the wall of the aorta at the preferred site. This difficulty can be approached in a number of ways. The first step is to grasp the needle close to the tip and again attempt to pass it through the wall. If this is performed too vigorously, the plaque may fracture and this may result in tearing of the wall or dissection of the plaque so as to occlude the lumen. The second approach is to seek, with the tip of the needle, a softer part of the wall in a *deeper* plane (Fig. 18.1 which shows an end-to-side anastomosis). This results in incorporation of more of the wall in the suture line. If less of the wall is taken, there is a substantial risk of the plaque breaking and the suture tearing through. Several of these deep sutures may be necessary (as shown in the figure) before the end of the plaque is reached when the sutures can be placed at the preferred depth. If neither of these measures can be used, one successful method is to take a sharp-pointed towel clip and use it to make holes in the wall of the aorta through which sutures can be passed. Another method is to place the sutures only through the adventitial layers of the aortic wall, external to the calcification. These sutures must be placed very gently to avoid tearing this thin tissue.

Figure 18.2 shows how calcification at the aortic bifurcation is dealt with. The calcified plaque is indicated by the area like a tongue extending into the aorta. Sutures are placed in the lumen beyond the plaque and emerge into the lumen of the aneurysm. The first suture of the second side is a mattress suture on the prosthesis: the needle on the right-hand side of Figure 18.2a is passed from outside the prosthesis to the inside. It is then placed into the lumen of the right common iliac artery in a similar manner to the suture on the left.

Endarterectomy should be undertaken infrequently. Attempts at endarterectomy may result in the calcified plaque, which may be the whole circumference of the aorta, tearing the adventitia. This may be impossible to repair. The formal attempt to perform endarterectomy on a segment of the aorta should be distinguished from the removal of loose atheromatous debris, although, even in these circumstances, the effects of weakening the aortic wall must be remembered. The major risk is difficulty in achieving haemostasis at the suture line rather than any possible risk of late false aneurysm.

Another point of possible damage is the site of application of the clamp. Closing the clamp on a heavily calcified aorta may result in fracture of plaques which lacerate the wall. Figure 18.3 shows the mechanism. The distal part of the plaque is between the jaws of the clamp. The proximal part is shown perforating the wall of the aorta. The clamp occludes the hole so that bleeding may not occur until the clamp is released, when serious bleeding is seen to be coming from above the suture line. This situation illustrated in Figure 18.4a may be difficult to retrieve. Bleeding should be controlled by digital pressure while the aorta is dissected to allow a clamp to be applied safely above the site of injury. If, as is usual, the initial clamp was close to the renal arteries, the aorta must be dissected to allow safe placement of a clamp above the tear. Supracoeliac clamping (see p. 144) is the preferred option. Once the bleeding has been controlled the site of injury is inspected. It may be possible to repair the laceration by placing one or more fine (5/0) sutures transversely across the defect (Fig. 18.4b). If the laceration is extensive it may be necessary to redo the anastomosis at a higher level where the wall is softer.

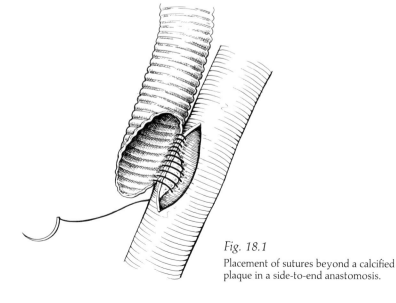

Fig. 18.1
Placement of sutures beyond a calcified plaque in a side-to-end anastomosis.

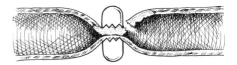

Fig. 18.3
Mechanism by which plaque tears arterial wall.

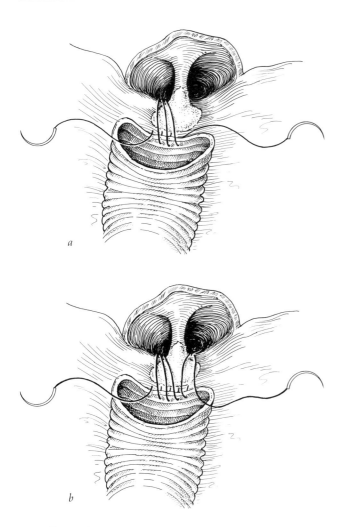

Fig. 18.2
Calcification at aortic bifurcation; placement of sutures.

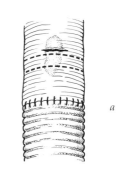

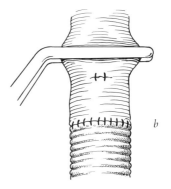

Fig. 18.4
(a) Position of tear. Plaque stippled; position of clamp indicated by dotted line. (b) Clamp placed above defect which is sutured.

OTHER ANEURYSMS OF THE LOWER LIMB

Chapter 19

Iliac artery

Introduction

Dilatation of the common iliac artery is present in about 20% of patients with abdominal aortic aneurysm. Its management has been discussed on page 134. Rarely, the patient may present with an aneurysm of the common or internal iliac artery without significant abdominal aortic aneurysm. These represent about 2% of abdominal aneurysms (Richardson & Greenfield 1988). The natural history of these aneurysms is uncertain but the incidence of rupture appears to be high because about 50–70% of cases present as ruptured aneurysm. Aneurysms of the external iliac artery are exceedingly rare and are almost always associated with other aneurysms.

CLINICAL FEATURES

Prior to rupture, these aneurysms are usually detected incidentally during the course of some other investigation or examination. Multiple aneurysms are present in 23–72% of patients. A mass may be felt on abdominal or pelvic examination in 70% of cases (Richardson & Greenfield 1988). It may be difficult to determine if the pulsatile mass is in the iliac artery or from a tortuous aneurysmal aorta. Internal iliac artery aneurysms are often larger when detected than aneurysms of the common iliac artery. Isolated aneurysms may cause pain from expansion or symptoms from pressure on neighbouring organs. These include bladder, bowel and ureter. Lumbosacral nerve roots may also be compressed and pain may be referred to the leg or buttock. Pain may result from renal distension from ureteric obstruction, and there have been occasional reports of acute iliofemoral venous thrombosis as the presenting feature. The diagnosis may be made on pelvic or rectal examination. Following rupture, the blood loss is usually substantially less than in ruptured abdominal aortic aneurysm and thus the features of circulatory collapse are less prominent. This can result in delay in diagnosis. There is a significant mortality from ruptured iliac aneurysm.

DIAGNOSTIC TESTS

A computed tomographic (CT) scan is the test which will give the most information about the aneurysm and the state of the adjacent vessels.

INDICATIONS FOR OPERATION

Symptomatic aneurysms should be repaired before rupture occurs. The decision is more difficult in the case of asymptomatic common iliac aneurysms. The decision in abdominal aortic aneurysm is discussed elsewhere (p. 134) and the principles relating to abdominal aortic aneurysms can be applied to patients with iliac artery aneurysm. The available evidence on the natural history suggests that repair should be advised in aneurysms of the iliac arteries > 3.0 cm in diameter.

PREOPERATIVE CARE

The preoperative preparation should be as for an abdominal aortic aneurysm because it may not be possible to repair the iliac aneurysm without clamping the aorta.

OPERATION

Oblique extraperitoneal approach
A midline incision is suitable but an extraperitoneal approach may be used if the surgeon is confident that it will not be necessary to dissect the iliac artery on the opposite side. The incision begins at the lateral edge of the rectus sheath, halfway between the pubic symphysis and the umbilicus, and continues laterally, parallel to the inguinal ligament (Fig. 19.1a, b). The fibres of the external oblique muscle are split and the internal oblique and transversus abdominus muscles are divided. The transversalis fascia is divided in the lateral part of the wound because it is less attached to the peritoneum than in the medial part. The hand is inserted into the iliac fossa in the extraperitoneal plane and the peritoneum swept medially. This dissection continues until the aortic bifurcation is reached (Fig. 19.2). The ureter, which crosses the bifurcation of

the common iliac artery, is seen as it is swept forward with the peritoneum. The peritoneum is covered with a damp pack and the blade of a fixed retractor inserted over it. A second blade is placed against the iliac crest. This approach gives excellent exposure of the external and distal common iliac arteries. The figure shows the limit of the proximal dissection which can be achieved comfortably using this approach. If exposure of the aortic bifurcation is required, the incision may be extended medially by dividing the anterior and posterior layers of the rectus sheath and retracting or dividing the muscle. However, in a large patient, exposure of the aortic bifurcation, especially from the right side, may be difficult, and if this is likely to be necessary an alternative approach is recommended.

Pararectus extraperitoneal approach
The incision (Fig. 19.3) begins 5 cm above the pubic tubercle and continues proximally about 2.5 cm lateral to the lateral edge of the rectus sheath to a point lateral to and just above the umbilicus. The muscles are divided in the line of the incision. The transversalis fascia is divided and separated carefully from the peritoneum. Medially, the fascia and peritoneum may be closely adherent and it is very easy to damage the peritoneum. If a hole is made it should be repaired at this stage. The peritoneum is dissected from lateral to medial as described in the previous section. This incision is more destructive of muscle and will denervate sections of the rectus abdominus muscle. The exposure obtained is similar to that illustrated in Figure 19.2. However, it has the great advantage that it can be extended proximally as far as is necessary to obtain control of the aorta and this is a major safety factor. This incision should not be used if there has been a previous midline or ipsilateral paramedian incision.

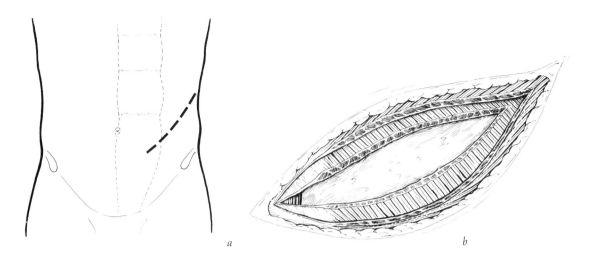

Fig. 19.1
Oblique extraperitoneal approach showing skin incision and muscle layers in incision.

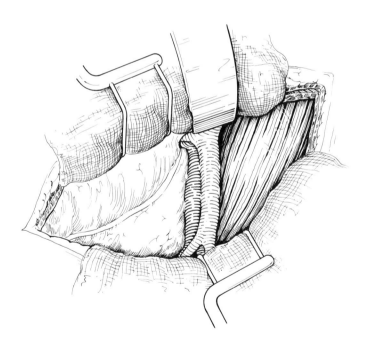

Fig. 19.2
Exposure of left iliac vessels and ureter.

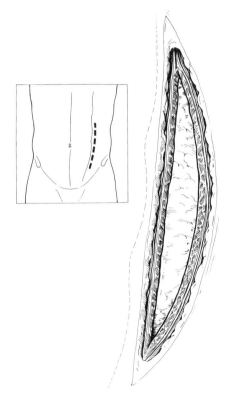

Fig. 19.3
Vertical pararectus incision.

Common iliac artery aneurysm—no prior aortic surgery

If an abdominal aortic aneurysm is found during preoperative evaluation the operation should proceed as described on page 122.

If the aneurysm is confined to the iliac artery a graft can be placed from proximal to distal common iliac artery. More dissection in the region of the aortic bifurcation is necessary than in an elective abdominal aortic aneurysm because of the need to place a clamp behind the aorta (Fig. 19.4). This dissection should proceed with great care because of the risk of injury to the left common iliac vein. It is desirable to place a clamp in this position in order to maintain the arterial supply to the opposite limb. The presence of a calcified plaque at the bifurcation may make it unsafe to apply a clamp in this way. In this event, the lower aorta and the opposite common iliac artery should be formally dissected and it may be necessary to place an aortobi-iliac graft. After dissection of the external and internal iliac arteries as described on page 135, the vessels are clamped. The aneurysm is opened through a 'T' incision in its anterior wall and an end-to-end anastomosis fashioned using the inlay technique. A graft of 10–12 mm will usually be used. The distal anastomosis is performed using one of the methods described on page 136.

In some cases, particularly if the aneurysm has ruptured, it may be easier to oversew or staple the origin of the common iliac artery, ligate or staple the distal common iliac artery and perform a femoral crossover graft to restore the circulation to the limb and, by retrograde perfusion of the external iliac artery, to the pelvis (Fig. 19.5).

Common iliac artery aneurysm following aortic aneurysm resection

The procedure to be performed depends on the anatomy of the previous reconstruction. Most commonly the common iliac aneurysm will be distal to an end-to-end anastomosis between graft and aorta (Fig. 19.6) and the origin of the common iliac artery will not be suitable for anastomosis as described in the preceding section. Dissection is likely to be difficult. The aortic graft must be dissected and controlled. The opposite iliac system must also be controlled. It may be easier to do this more distally by dissecting the external and internal iliac arteries because this region might not have been dissected previously and because it is further away from the major veins. Finally, the ipsilateral external and internal iliac arteries must be controlled. The ureters must be identified carefully. They will usually be densely adherent to the vessels and must be separated gently to allow adequate exposure. Extensive mobilization of the ureters should not be undertaken for fear of damaging their blood supply.

The preferred reconstruction is the insertion of an aortobi-iliac graft. The reasons are that it is likely to be very difficult to control the orifice of the ipsilateral iliac artery and there is a high probability that the opposite iliac artery will be abnormal. The aortic graft is transected and the lower segment removed. A new bifurcation graft is anastomosed end-to-end to the original graft. The distal ends are anastomosed to the iliac vessels in one of the ways described on page 136.

Occasionally, the anatomy will be as shown in Figure 19.7. In this case the original graft has been anastomosed to the external iliac artery and the origin of the common iliac artery closed at the time of the insertion of the original graft. The aneurysm is being filled by retrograde flow through the external and internal iliac artery. It is easy to exclude the common iliac aneurysm in these circumstances. If there is certain knowledge of the details of the previous operation, an extraperitoneal approach may be used. The ipsilateral limb of the graft is located and dissected without damage to the ureter, which is commonly densely adherent to its anterior surface. The external iliac artery is dissected from the lateral side distal to the anastomosis. The extent of the proximal dissection required depends on the need to preserve the internal iliac artery. If it is to be preserved, the distal common iliac artery must be dissected and ligated or stapled (see p. 137) at the proximal site shown in Figure 19.7. If it is not to be preserved, the external iliac artery is ligated proximal to the anastomosis at the distal site shown in Figure 19.7.

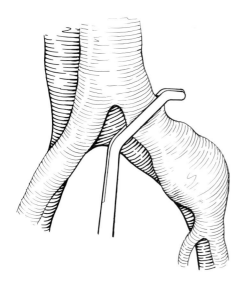

Fig. 19.4
Clamp across origin of left common iliac artery.

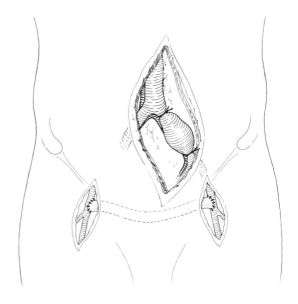

Fig. 19.5
Proximal and distal ligation of aneurysm and femoral cross-over graft.

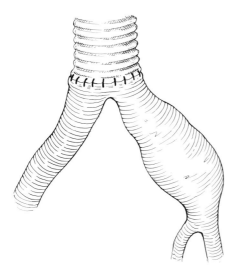

Fig. 19.6
Aneurysm distal to previous aortic graft.

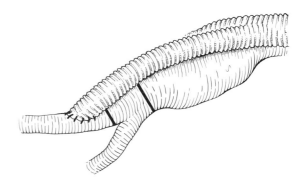

Fig. 19.7
Previous bypass to external iliac artery allows simple ligation above or below internal iliac artery origin.

Internal iliac artery aneurysm

These may be isolated lesions or associated with aortoiliac aneurysmal disease. Isolated aneurysms tend to be single, while aneurysms associated with aortoiliac aneurysmal disease are usually bilateral. False aneurysms following blunt trauma or operative injury have been reported. Operations on this lesion have been considered difficult because of the problem of obtaining distal control of the branches of the artery which arise deep in the pelvis and come from the lateral aspect of the aneurysm. These problems are lessened by the technique of repair from within the aneurysm described here. An oblique extraperitoneal approach is used (Fig. 19.1). The common and external iliac arteries are dissected and encircled after identification of the ureter. The external and common iliac arteries are clamped and the aneurysm opened along its medial wall. Laminated thrombus and atheromatous debris are removed. Back-bleeding which may be profuse will be seen to be coming from one to three major sources in the depth of the aneurysm cavity (Fig. 19.8). If the bleeding is profuse, balloon catheters should be introduced into these branches to occlude them. A cross-stitch is placed across the orifice, the balloon deflated and the catheter withdrawn before the suture is tied. If there is less bleeding, suction deep in the cavity may provide sufficient visibility to allow placement of the suture. Although these sutures are deep in the pelvis, suturing from within the lumen is the easiest and safest way of securing these vessels. Extensive dissection of the external surface of the aneurysm in order to place clamps across the branches is very difficult and there is a major risk of producing venous haemorrhage which may be difficult to control. There is no attempt to remove the aneurysm sac. The origin of the internal iliac artery is ligated or oversewn.

Preservation of the internal iliac artery

If both internal iliac arteries are occluded (or aneurysmal) and the inferior mesenteric artery has been occluded (either by atheroma or previous surgery), at least one of the internal iliac arteries should be repaired. This may be a very difficult technical exercise. The preferred method is to insert a short interposition graft of 8 mm diameter prosthesis. The distal anastomosis is performed first. The graft is placed within the aneurysm cavity and anastomosed around the orifices of the major branches in a manner analogous to that illustrated in Figure 11.5. The proximal end of the graft is anastomosed to a convenient point on the side of the common or external iliac artery.

False aneurysm of an aortoiliac anastomosis

These lesions are less common than after aortofemoral grafting but they are reported to have a high propensity for rupture (Treiman et al 1988). Asymptomatic lesions may be detected during investigation of abdominal symptoms, particularly by CT scanning. Aneurysms presenting late after surgery are unlikely to be infected (see discussion of femoral false aneurysms, p. 236). Surgical repair should be undertaken for significant aneurysms because of their inaccessibility for surveillance and the technical difficulty of dealing with them when they rupture.

An oblique extraperitoneal approach is used. The graft is located and clamped if the aneurysm is leaking. The external iliac artery is dissected and controlled.

The method of repair depends on the technique which has been used in the previous operation and the presence or absence of infection. If the false aneurysm presents years after the primary surgery, the prosthetic graft is well incorporated with fibrous tissue and there are no local signs of infection, local repair may be undertaken.

Prior end-to-end iliac anastomosis (Fig. 19.9a–c)

Clamps are applied and the aneurysm opened. Bleeding from the internal iliac artery is controlled by a balloon catheter in its lumen. This is safer than attempting to dissect the artery which has been dissected previously. Once control has been obtained, the graft at the anastomosis should be completely separated from the artery. If a direct repair is to be performed the graft is trimmed and a new piece of the same diameter anastomosed end to end. The distal common iliac artery is ligated (Fig. 19.9b), preserving the internal iliac artery if possible. The distal anastomosis is performed end to side to the external iliac artery. If there is doubt about the presence of infection the graft is clamped and divided and oversewn as close as possible to its bifurcation. Reconstruction is by a femorofemoral crossover graft as shown in Figure 19.5.

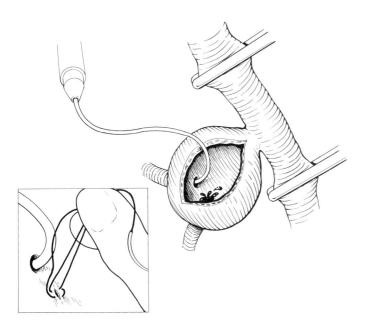

Fig. 19.8
Aneurysm of internal iliac artery; control of branches by
Fogarty catheter; suturing orifice from within lumen.

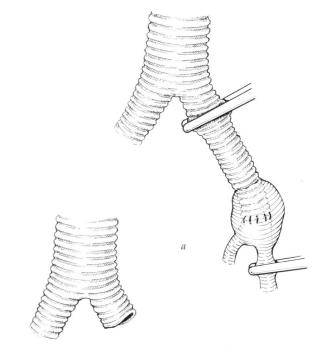

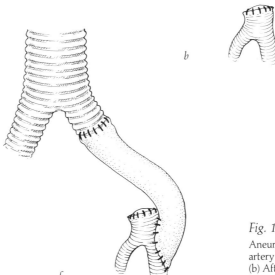

Fig. 19.9
Aneurysm at graft to common iliac
artery anastomosis. (a) Overall view.
(b) After excision of part of
graft. (c) Reconstruction.

Prior end-to-side anastomosis
(Fig. 19.10a–c)
If possible the external iliac artery
proximal to the anastomosis should be
dissected in order to control back-
bleeding from the internal iliac artery
and clamped before the aneurysm is
opened. In the absence of infection the
graft is separated and trimmed as
described above. The external iliac
artery is ligated distal and if possible
proximal to the internal iliac artery
(Fig. 19.10b). The distal anastomosis of
the new segment of graft may be to the
external iliac artery more distally or to
the common femoral artery.
Alternatively the graft may be ligated
and a femorofemoral crossover graft
performed.

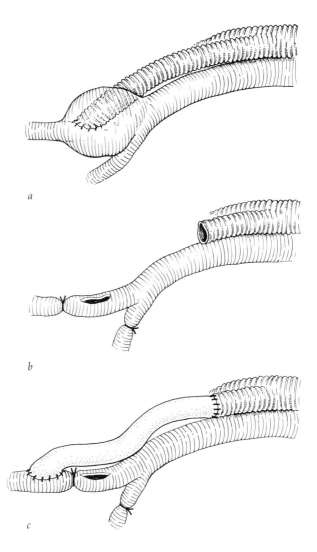

a

b

c

Fig. 19.10
Aneurysm at external iliac artery anastomosis. (a) Lateral view. (b) After excision of part of graft.
(c) Reconstruction.

REFERENCES

Perdue G D, Mittenthal M J, Smith R B III, Salam A A 1983 Aneurysms of
    the internal iliac artery. Surgery 93: 243–246
Richardson J W, Greenfield L J 1988 Natural history and management of
    iliac aneurysms. Journal of Vascular Surgery 8: 165–171
Treiman G S, Weaver F A, Cossman D V et al 1988 Anastomotic false
    aneurysms of the abdominal aorta and the iliac arteries. Journal of
    Vascular Surgery 8: 268–273

Chapter 20

Femoral artery

Classification

Aneurysm of the femoral arteries may be primary, resulting from atherosclerotic degeneration, or secondary to previous surgery or trauma. Infection is a frequent complication of secondary aneurysms and may be difficult to manage.

PRIMARY
'True', atherosclerotic aneurysm
    common femoral artery
    profunda femoris artery
    superficial femoral artery

SECONDARY
Anastomotic   infected or non-infected
Traumatic   infected or non-infected

(Anastomotic and traumatic aneurysms are considered in Section F, Chapter 23.)

ATHEROSCLEROTIC ANEURYSMS OF FEMORAL ARTERY

The normal upper limit for the diameter of the common femoral artery in male patients is approximately 1.5 cm and in females approximately 1.0 cm (Johnston et al 1991). Mild dilatation of the common femoral artery is frequent in patients with aneurysmal disease and aneurysms of the femoral artery are present in 3–7% of patients with abdominal aortic aneurysm (Dent et al 1972). Almost all patients who present with femoral aneurysms are male. Multiple aneurysms are present in 70–80% of patients with a femoral aneurysm. Bilateral aneurysms are present in 72%, and abdominal aortic aneurysm in 85–92% (Dent et al 1972, Graham et al 1980).

CLINICAL FEATURES

In patients whose only symptom is the presence of a mass, the natural history is benign with few serious complications occurring (Graham et al 1980). In the 60% who present with symptoms these may include rupture or painful expansion, thrombosis and large vessel or small vessel embolism. Ischaemia of the limb occurs in about 10% of cases.

DIAGNOSTIC TESTS

The diagnosis is made by palpation of the mass. The patient should be evaluated carefully for other aneurysms which may have a higher priority for treatment. Careful abdominal examination should be supplemented by ultrasound examination. The popliteal fossae should also be examined carefully for aneurysms.

It is conventional to perform angiography to display the anatomy of the aneurysm and, particularly, its outflow vessels. Duplex ultrasound can provide this information and should replace angiography as the investigation of choice.

INDICATIONS FOR OPERATION

In many cases the aneurysm is too small to justify surgery. However, if the aneurysm is greater than 2.5 cm in diameter or if there is a history suggesting rapid expansion or if embolism occurs, operation should be undertaken.

PREOPERATIVE CARE

Surgery on these lesions is usually well tolerated by the patient. After assessing the cardiorespiratory fitness of the patient for surgery, the most important preoperative step is to look for abdominal aortic aneurysm.

OPERATION

The major factor affecting the conduct of the operation is the anatomy of the aneurysm and whether it involves the superficial femoral artery or the profunda femoris artery.

The common femoral artery is approached through a standard vertical incision. The superficial tissues are dissected from the aneurysm. The common femoral artery should be controlled as it emerges from beneath the inguinal ligament. There is usually room for this to be carried out below the inguinal ligament although the ligament may need to be mobilized and retracted (see Fig. 20.1). The deep circumflex iliac and deep epigastric branches of the external iliac artery should be sought deliberately and

controlled with 3/0 silk slings. The external iliac artery is almost always normal. Rarely, it will be necessary to expose and control the external iliac artery as described on page 237.

The superficial femoral artery is dissected distal to the aneurysm and a sling placed around it. The aneurysm is freed from surrounding tissues by dissecting distally from the common femoral artery and proximally from the superficial femoral artery (Fig. 20.2a).

If the profunda femoris artery is not involved, its origin is dissected and encircled with a tape. If the profunda femoris artery is aneurysmal, its wall must be dissected until normal artery is reached. The large veins crossing inferior to the artery, deep to the superficial femoral artery, should be dissected carefully and ligated (Fig. 20.2b) or oversewn. The aneurysm may extend down to the first major branch of the profunda femoris artery.

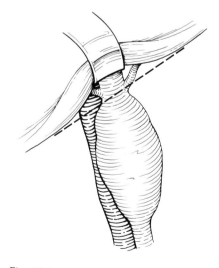

Fig. 20.1
Retraction of inguinal ligament to display neck of femoral aneurysm.

Complete dissection of the inflow and outflow is preferred to a policy of limited dissection with balloon catheter occlusion of the distal vessels because the dissection is usually not difficult and the surgeon is operating in familiar territory. In addition, distal dissection, particularly of the profunda femoris artery, will need to be undertaken to perform the anastomosis and it is preferable to perform this dissection in a dry field before opening the aneurysm rather than in more difficult conditions later in the operation.

The reconstruction necessary depends on the anatomy of the aneurysm.

Common femoral artery only involved

Clamps are applied to the common femoral artery as close to the inguinal ligament as possible and to the superficial femoral artery and profunda femoris artery distal to the aneurysm. The aneurysm is opened vertically along its length. It is transected at its neck and at its lower end the openings of the superficial femoral artery and the profunda femoris artery are preserved as a common orifice (Fig. 20.3). The wall of the aneurysm may be excised but areas adjacent to important structures like the femoral vein and nerve need not be disturbed.

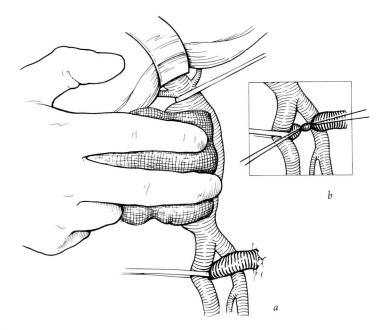

Fig. 20.2
(a) Dissection of aneurysm of common femoral artery. (b) Ligation of profunda femoris vein.

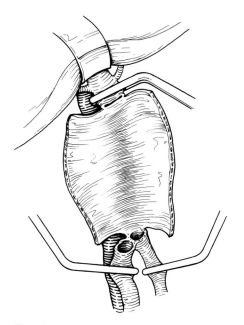

Fig. 20.3
Common femoral aneurysm prepared for anastomosis.

A graft of appropriate diameter (commonly 8–10 mm) is chosen. Knitted Dacron (which should be pre-clotted before heparinization of the patient) or PTFE are appropriate. The graft is anastomosed end to end to the defect in the common femoral artery using a continuous 5/0 monofilament suture. The proximal end of the graft is cut transversely. The distal end may need to be divided obliquely to encompass the orifices of both the distal vessels (Fig. 20.4).

Common femoral artery and superficial femoral artery involved
(Fig. 20.5a)

As the wall of the aneurysm is resected, a rim of wall is left around the orifice of the profunda femoris artery. This facilitates the anastomosis between the graft and the profunda femoris artery. After performance of the proximal anastomosis, a hole is cut in the back of the graft where it will overlie the orifice of the profunda femoris artery. The orifice of the profunda femoris artery is sutured to this defect as shown in Figure 20.5b before the distal anastomosis between graft and superficial femoral artery is performed.

Common femoral artery and profunda femoris artery involved
(Fig. 20.6a)

As the aneurysm is resected, the superficial femoral artery is transected at its origin. It is easier if the most difficult anastomosis, that between graft and profunda femoris artery, is performed first. An end-to-end anastomosis is performed between these two vessels. The anastomosis between common femoral artery and graft is performed next and, finally, the end of the superficial femoral artery is anastomosed to a hole cut in the side of the graft (Fig. 20.6b). (This latter step is omitted if the superficial femoral artery is occluded.)

All three vessels involved

The reconstruction is similar to that in Figure 20.6b. After the profunda femoris artery and common femoral artery anastomoses are complete, the clamps can be released and blood flow restored to the limb. A further segment of prosthesis is anastomosed to the end of the superficial femoral artery and, finally, to the side of the graft between the common femoral artery and the profunda femoris artery (Fig. 20.7).

Aneurysm of the superficial femoral artery

Isolated aneurysm of the superficial femoral artery is a rare lesion which often presents in frail elderly male patients. It presents with an expanding mass in the thigh which is tender. There may be bruising indicating extravasation of blood. The distal circulation is usually intact. Ultrasound examination may provide sufficient information to allow planning of surgery by demonstrating non-dilated segments proximal and distal to the aneurysm. However, in most cases angiography will be performed to delineate the lesion.

Replacement of the aneurysm is usually straightforward. The superficial femoral artery is controlled at a convenient site above the aneurysm and, depending on the lower extent of the aneurysm, distal control is obtained by dissecting either the distal superficial femoral artery or the popliteal artery. There are not usually any significant branches from the artery at this level, so that back-bleeding from collateral branches is not a problem. The graft used may be either long saphenous or a prosthesis of Dacron or PTFE. In performing an emergency procedure on a frail patient it is quicker to use a prosthetic graft. In addition, if the ends of the artery are dilated the long saphenous vein might not be wide enough.

On rare occasions true atherosclerotic aneurysms may arise in a vein graft. The probable mechanism is atherosclerotic degeneration in the graft. They present as a mass in the thigh in the line of the graft and are treated by excision and replacement of the affected segment.

RESULTS

The mortality and morbidity are low. Patients who were asymptomatic before operation can expect to remain free of symptoms. However, symptoms of various sorts will persist in about half of those presenting with symptoms.

REFERENCES

Cutler B S, Darling R C 1973 Surgical management of arteriosclerotic femoral aneurysms. Surgery 74: 764–773
Dent T L, Lindenauer S M, Ernst C B, Fry W J 1972 Multiple arteriosclerotic arterial aneurysms. Archives of Surgery 105: 338–344
Graham L M, Zelenock G B, Whitehouse W M et al 1980 Clinical significance of arteriosclerotic femoral artery aneurysms. Archives of Surgery 115: 502–507
Johnston K W, Rutherford R B, Tilson M D, Shah D M, Hollier L, Stanley J C 1991 Suggested standards for reporting on arterial aneurysms. Journal of Vascular Surgery 13: 444–450

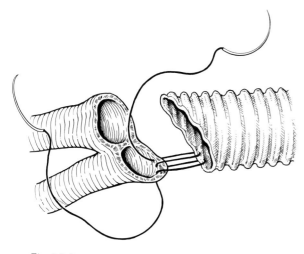

Fig. 20.4
Detail of beginning anastomosis.

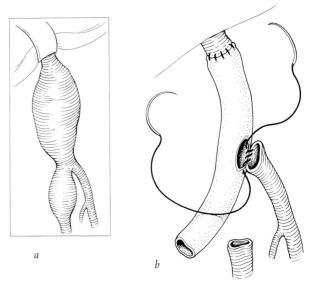

a   b

Fig. 20.5
Aneurysm of common femoral and superficial femoral arteries.
(a) Anatomy. (b) Reconstruction of profunda femoris artery.

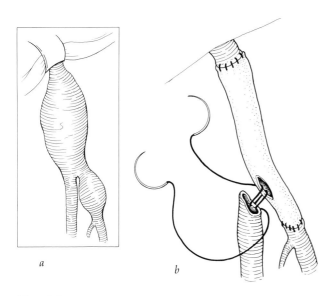

a   b

Fig. 20.6
Aneurysm of common femoral artery and profunda femoris artery.
(a) Anatomy. (b) Reconstruction of profunda femoris artery.

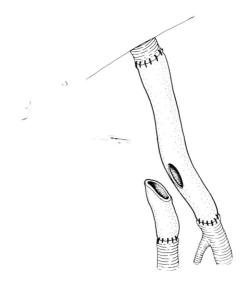

Fig. 20.7
Interposition graft between prosthesis
and superficial femoral artery.

Chapter 21

Popliteal artery

Introduction

The popliteal artery is the commonest site of aneurysm formation apart from the abdominal aorta and accounts for about 70% of peripheral aneurysms. Popliteal aneurysms are frequently associated with aortic aneurysm. It is estimated that popliteal aneurysms occur in 8% of patients with abdominal aortic aneurysm (Guvendik et al 1980) and abdominal aortic aneurysm will be found in about one-third to one-half of patients with popliteal aneurysm. Popliteal aneurysms are frequently bilateral: estimates of the incidence range from one-third to two-thirds. Thus, examination of the popliteal arteries is an essential part of the clinical examination of patients with abdominal aortic aneurysm and vice versa. Popliteal aneurysms occur most commonly in patients between the ages of 50 and 80 years and are 30 times more common in male patients.

Almost all popliteal aneurysms are atherosclerotic in origin and many patients have the risk factors for atherosclerosis, especially smoking and hypertension.

CLINICAL FEATURES

Asymptomatic patients
Popliteal aneurysms are often symptomless and detected during routine examination. In other cases they may present as a mass behind the knee which has to be differentiated from synovial (Baker's) cysts. Spontaneous thrombosis of the aneurysm may not cause any symptoms.

Chronic symptoms
Patients presenting with an occluded aneurysm may present with chronic ischaemia. The symptoms may include intermittent claudication or limb-threatening ischaemia with rest pain and/or gangrene. Less commonly (8%, Vermillion et al 1981) patients may present with symptoms of pressure on the adjacent nerve or vein (Fig. 21.1).

A small group of patients present with microembolism to the skin of the foot. This may produce small skin infarcts or gangrene of a toe. The condition is often mistaken for a connective tissue disorder.

Acute symptoms
Acute ischaemia
Acute severe limb ischaemia is a common presentation of popliteal aneurysm and represents a serious threat to the survival of the limb. The diagnosis may be made by palpating the aneurysm or a contralateral popliteal aneurysm. However, in many cases, the presence of an aneurysm is not suspected until the artery has been explored or the lumen revealed following thrombolysis. Thrombosis of the aneurysm may occur after a period during which the calf vessels have become occluded progressively by embolus from the aneurysm.

Rupture
This is uncommon, with an incidence of about 3% of the major complications.

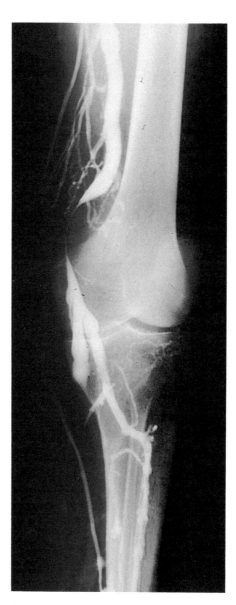

Fig. 21.1
Compression of popliteal vein.

DIAGNOSTIC TESTS

1.   If there is doubt about the presence of the aneurysm or if differentiation from other masses in the popliteal fossa is necessary, ultrasound examination is the method of choice: it is quick, painless, cheap and accurate.
2.   If the aneurysm is of a size that surgery is indicated, or if the patient presents with symptoms of distal ischaemia, angiography (Fig. 21.2) should be performed. This will show the extent of occlusion of the arteries of the calf, and display the anatomy of the arteries so that appropriate surgery can be planned. Angiography, if performed as the primary diagnostic modality, may fail to demonstrate the aneurysm in about 10% of cases.

Various patterns of aneurysms are seen. In some, the wall is smooth and the dilatation localized to the popliteal artery. In others (Fig. 21.2), the popliteal aneurysm is the lower end of a process which involves much of the superficial femoral artery.

INDICATIONS FOR OPERATION

Asymptomatic patients
Studies of the natural history of untreated aneurysms have produced conflicting evidence. On the one hand, an annual incidence of limb-threatening complications of 10% has been reported (Anton et al 1986, Vermillion et al 1981). On the other hand, others have quoted a much lower risk (e.g. Schellack et al 1987). The situation is made more difficult because of the good results obtained from operation in asymptomatic patients compared with the 20–30% chance of amputation when acute complications develop.

In asymptomatic patients, operation is advised in a fit patient with an aneurysm of 2.0 cm or greater diameter. Patients with smaller lesions, or who are less fit, or in whom the aneurysm is one of many, may be treated expectantly with follow-up by means of regular ultrasound examination. However, it has been suggested that size is not a strong predictor of complications (Vermillion et al 1981). Difficult situations will be encountered. An obvious example is the patient with an abdominal aortic aneurysm with bilateral significant popliteal aneurysms. It is quite difficult, when counselling him about his abdominal aortic aneurysm operation, to say that he will need two subsequent procedures for treatment of his popliteal aneurysms. These patients often have generalized arteriomegaly which has been reported to carry a high risk of complications (Schellack et al 1987).

Chronic ischaemia

In many cases the presence of the aneurysm is less important than the state of the calf arteries which may also be occluded from repeated embolism from the popliteal aneurysm. This means that a distal bypass graft to the crural vessels may be necessary to save the limb. The outcome is clearly less favourable in patients with occluded calf arteries (Anton et al 1986).

Acute ischaemia

This is the presenting feature in about 25% of patients. Thrombolytic therapy is the preferred method of initial treatment. Thrombolysis will remove thrombus from the calf vessels and may restore the blood flow. Elective surgery is then performed to bypass the aneurysm. In some cases, occlusion of the aneurysm may follow an acute myocardial infarction. Thrombolytic therapy may be life saving in these patients by avoiding the risks of urgent surgery. In this group of patients anticoagulant therapy is given for 6 months before undertaking elective surgery.

With rapid expansion of the aneurysm or bruising of the tissues indicating that

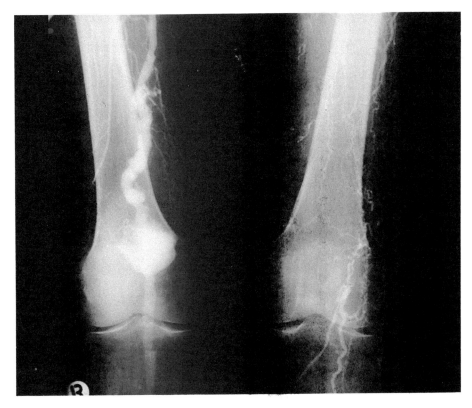

Fig. 21.2
Popliteal aneurysm. Occluded aneurysm on opposite side.

rupture has occurred, urgent operation is required.

In patients with aneurysms at multiple sites and without acute symptoms, an abdominal aortic aneurysm has the highest priority for treatment because rupture may result in the death of the patient. A popliteal aneurysm should be treated next because of its potential to threaten the viability of the limb. A femoral aneurysm has the lowest priority.

OPERATION

Bypass of popliteal aneurysm

The aneurysm may be approached through either a medial or a posterior approach to the popliteal artery. It is safer to bypass the aneurysm than to attempt to resect it because of the risks of damage to surrounding structures (especially veins) during resection.

Medial approach

This is used most commonly. It is the most familiar because it is used regularly in femorodistal bypass surgery. The whole length of the popliteal artery can be displayed by dividing the muscles and tendons on the medial side, namely sartorius, gracilis and semitendinosus in the more superficial plane and the medial head of gastrocnemius in the deeper plane. This will be necessary when dealing with a ruptured aneurysm. However, in most cases, it is not necessary to expose the whole length of the aneurysm. The popliteal artery approach below can be combined with a separate incision to approach the lower part of the superficial femoral artery or the upper part of the popliteal artery. If there is coexistent stenotic disease of the superficial femoral artery, a conventional femoropopliteal bypass can be performed. The upper and lower parts of the artery are exposed before the proximal anastomosis is performed.

Proximal dissection. The proximal end of the bypass graft is placed on a convenient segment of the lower superficial femoral artery or the upper part of the popliteal artery. Exposure of the superficial femoral artery is easier. The incision marked 'A' in Figure 21.3 is made over the sartorius muscle from the region of the adductor tubercle and extending 7–10 cm proximally. The fascia over the sartorius muscle is divided and the muscle retracted posteriorly. After dividing the deeper layer of fascia, a self-retaining retractor is inserted, the upper part of the

popliteal fossa is entered and the adipose/areolar tissue dissected. The sartorius muscle is retracted. The gastrocnemius muscle is visible in the distal part of the wound (Fig. 21.4). The pulse in the artery can be felt and the artery is freed from its attachments for a length of 3–4 cm and encircled with tapes as shown. There are often small veins around the artery. These may be ligated. Care should be taken to preserve branches arising from the lower part of the artery (one is shown in Fig. 21.4) as these may be important sources of collateral blood supply.

Distal dissection. The skin incision ('B' in Fig. 21.3) is made on the medial aspect of the calf over the long saphenous vein, approximately 1 cm posterior to the medial border of the tibia, starting at the level of the popliteal crease and extending distally for 10–12 cm. The vein and the saphenous nerve, which is close to the vein, are preserved. Major tributaries of the long saphenous vein may be ligated, but it is not necessary to mobilize the main vessel because the most proximal segment of vein is the conduit of choice for a bypass graft.

The deep fascia is incised throughout the length of the incision close to the tibia. This incision swings posteriorly in its upper part as the semitendinosus tendon is encountered, unless it is necessary to expose the whole length of the popliteal artery, in which case the

proximal and distal incisions are joined directly. The gastrocnemius muscle is displaced posteriorly by a self-retaining retractor in the lower part of the wound (Fig. 21.5). The soleus muscle can be seen anteroinferiorly and the semitendinosus tendon is shown in the anterosuperior part of the wound. After dissecting some loose adipose/areolar tissue in the popliteal fossa, the popliteal neurovascular bundle can be seen and felt in the bottom of the wound. Inferiorly, this bundle passes deep to the arch of the soleus muscle. The tibial nerve lies medial and posterior in the bundle at this level. It is not always seen, but should be displaced posteriorly if necessary. The artery is hidden from view by the veins which are usually both medial and lateral to the artery. While maintaining gentle traction on the medial vein, the lateral vein is separated from the artery by sharp dissection with scissors close to the artery. When a plane has been established, dissection takes place between the medial vein and the artery.

The insert shows the development of the plane between the artery and the veins which tend to surround it. Angled forceps and tape can be placed around the artery at this level and an adequate length of artery freed of its attachments. Dissection of the veins from the artery can be quite difficult. Inadvertent injury to the veins is best avoided by keeping the dissection as close as possible to the wall of the artery. In the more distal part, the artery may be encircled by

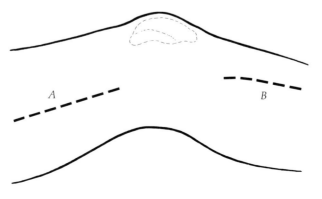

Fig. 21.3
Medial view of leg showing sites for incisions.

veins. In particular, the anterior tibial vein crosses the medial side of the popliteal artery at the level of the origin of the anterior tibial artery which is at the level of the soleal arch.

The dissection should be clear of the lower end of the aneurysm at this level. More exposure distally can be obtained by dissecting the artery down to the soleal arch and, if necessary, dividing the arch and separating the upper part of the muscle from the tibia. This is conveniently achieved by passing an index finger beneath the arch and cutting the muscle close to the tibia with sharp dissection or diathermy (Fig. 21.6). Further distal dissection can be carried out close to the artery, taking care to ligate any encircling branches of the veins (Fig. 21.7). This shows the divided fibres of soleus retracted in the distal part of the wound. The anterior tibial artery can be seen passing deeply in the anterior part of the wound. The anterior tibial vein has been divided and oversewn. The tibioperoneal trunk is visible at the level of the distal retractor. Occasionally more distal exposure of the tibial vessels is required. Details of these exposures is beyond the scope of this account (see Bell 1991).

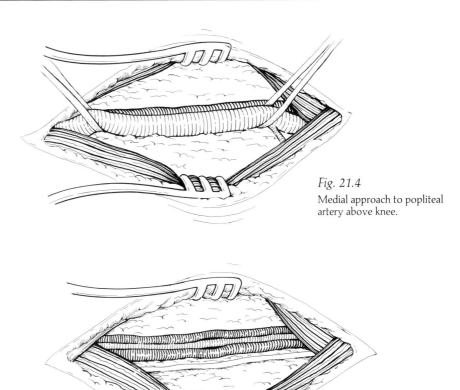

Fig. 21.4
Medial approach to popliteal artery above knee.

Fig. 21.5
Medial approach to popliteal artery below knee. Neurovascular bundle exposed. Beginning of separation of popliteal veins from artery.

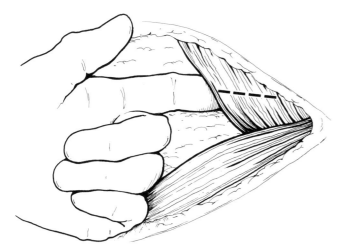

Fig. 21.6
Enlargement of incision by dividing attachment of soleus muscle close to tibia.

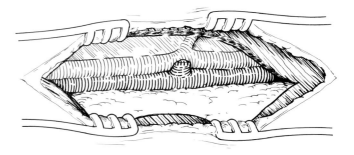

Fig. 21.7
Anterior tibial vein ligated showing origin of anterior tibial artery.

Anastomoses. The upper anastomosis is performed first. Traction on the tapes brings the popliteal artery into the more superficial part of the wound and facilitates the anastomosis. A side–end anastomosis (Fig. 4.7) is performed to a reversed saphenous vein graft taken preferably from the upper part of the long saphenous vein from the same limb. Figure 4.8 shows the placement of sutures before tightening the threads ('parachute' technique). Four to eight sutures may be placed before tightening. Once the anastomosis has been completed and haemostasis achieved, the graft is tunnelled deep to the gastrocnemius muscle into the popliteal fossa and anastomosed end to side to the popliteal artery prepared as described above (see Fig. 21.8). The distal segment of the superficial femoral artery and the popliteal artery proximal to the anastomosis are ligated or oversewn and the patency of the reconstruction checked by angiography (Fig. 21.9).

Posterior approach

This approach is suitable if the limits of the aneurysm are defined clearly on arteriography and the tibioperoneal trunk is patent. It is used less often because of its unfamiliarity and because it is necessary to be certain of the limits of the dissection that will be required before this approach is used. If pressure on nerve or vein is causing symptoms, this approach allows decompression of the aneurysm.

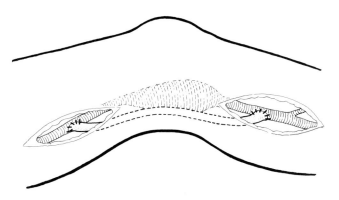

Fig. 21.8
View of completed bypass from medial approach.

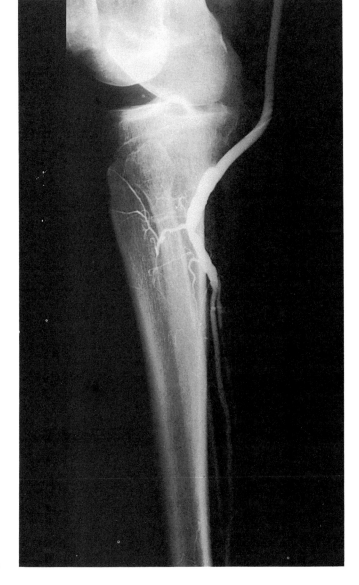

Fig. 21.9
Operative angiogram.

With the patient prone, the knee is flexed 10° by a sandbag under the foot. An 'S'-shaped incision is made in the popliteal fossa (Fig. 21.10). The horizontal limb of the 'S' is in the popliteal skin crease. The upper limb is placed medially over the adductor region and the lower limb passes down the lateral side of the fossa. The short saphenous vein is encountered and the sural nerve will be found deep to the deep fascia (Fig. 21.11). The popliteal artery is sought in the proximal end of the incision. It is dissected and encircled. This dissection may be difficult and require strong retraction of the semimembranosus and semitendinosus muscles medially and the biceps femoris laterally. The common peroneal nerve in the lateral part of the wound must be protected. The tibial nerve is superficial to the artery and must be separated with care. The artery is dissected in a similar fashion in the lower part of the popliteal fossa. It may be necessary to divide tributaries of the popliteal vein to gain adequate exposure but it is not necessary to completely separate the vein from the artery (Fig. 21.12). Access to the distal tibioperoneal trunk is poor. When the artery has been controlled, the aneurysm may be bypassed without opening the sac or, preferably, a graft may be inserted using an inlay technique analogous to that used for abdominal aortic aneurysm (Fig. 21.13). Branches which are bleeding may be controlled from within the sac. The redundant wall of the aneurysm may be excised but total excision is unnecessary.

Hunterian ligation
This procedure, in which the femoral artery is ligated proximal to the first major geniculate branch, still has a small place in a frail patient in whom the aneurysm is enlarging or causing pressure symptoms. The ligature is placed in the position of the inferior sling shown in Figure 21.4.

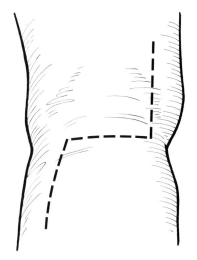

Fig. 21.10
Incision for posterior approach to popliteal artery.

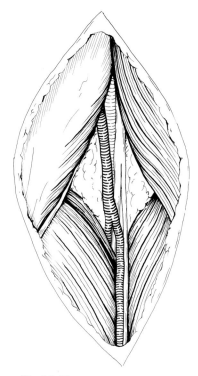

Fig. 21.11
Superficial dissection of popliteal fossa.

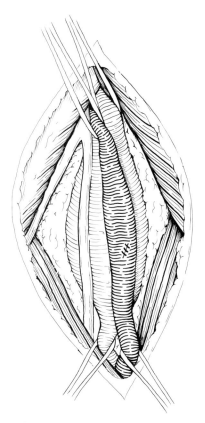

Fig. 21.12
Deep dissection of popliteal fossa.

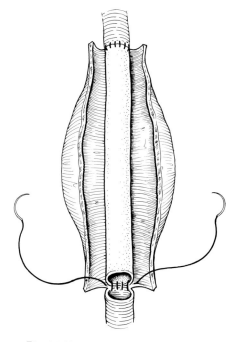

Fig. 21.13
Inlay graft being anastomosed end-to-end.

RESULTS

The reported postoperative course following aneurysm surgery suggests that the reconstructions are more durable than when performed for occlusive disease (Anton et al 1986, Vermillion et al 1981). This may reflect larger arteries and/or better run-off vessels, although this latter criterion does not always apply. By this view elective surgery is advised in most cases. However, there is sufficient uncertainty about the natural history of untreated aneurysm to justify a selective approach to surgery in asymptomatic patients. Added to the general and local complications of surgery, there is a small incidence of recurrence either proximal or distal to the reconstructed segment.

In patients with chronic ischaemia, the outcome will be largely influenced by the state of the calf arteries, being worse in those with occluded vessels (Anton et al 1986). Following surgery for acute ischaemia, the limb is lost in about 30–40% of cases (Vermillion et al 1981, Whitehouse et al 1983).

REFERENCES

Anton G E, Hertzer N R, Beven E G, O'Hara P J, Krajewski L P 1986
    Surgical management of popliteal aneurysms. Journal of Vascular Surgery
    3: 125–134
Bell P R F 1991 Arterial surgery of the lower limb. Churchill Livingstone,
    Edinburgh, pp 153–182
Guvendik K, Bloor K, Charlesworth D 1980 Popliteal aneurysm: sinister
    harbinger of sudden catastrophe. British Journal of Surgery 67: 294–296
Schellack J, Smith R B, Perdue G D 1987 Non-operative management of
    selected popliteal aneurysms. Archives of Surgery 122: 372–375
Vermillion B D, Kimmins S A, Pace W G, Evans W E 1981 A review of one
    hundred and forty-seven popliteal aneurysms with long-term follow-up.
    Surgery 90: 1009–1014

INFECTION AND FALSE ANEURYSM

Chapter 22

Aortic infection and aortoenteric fistula

DEFINITIONS

This group includes a variety of conditions in which there may be infection of the aorta and surrounding tissues or a communication between the intestine and the aorta or an aortic graft, with or without haemorrhage.

The terms used are defined as follows.

Primary infected aneurysm. These may result from primary infections of the wall of the aorta, infection of an aneurysm from a source of bacteraemia or direct spread from an adjacent septic focus. There has not been previous aortic surgery performed.

Graft infection. Bacteria present and multiplying in the tissues contiguous with a prosthesis.

Anastomotic false aneurysm. Aneurysmal dilatation of an anastomosis due to partial separation of the suture line. The lesion may be infected or not infected.

Aortoenteric fistula. A communication between the lumen of the aorta and the lumen of the duodenum.

Paraprosthetic fistula. A communication between the lumen of the duodenum and the wall of an aortic prosthesis. This is sometimes included as a type of aortoenteric fistula. Note that, strictly speaking, it is not a fistula because there is no communication between the lumen of two viscera.

Figure 22.1 demonstrates the relationships between the various conditions.

PRIMARY INFECTED ANEURYSM

This is a rare presentation of abdominal aortic aneurysm. There may be a source for the sepsis such as drug abuse or bacterial endocarditis. There is usually evidence of severe sepsis which may be acute or subacute in its presentation. Blood cultures are positive in only

about 50%, presumably because most patients have received antibiotics which suppress the growth of bacteria. The sudden appearance of an aneurysm or the enlargement of an abdominal aortic aneurysm accompanied by signs of sepsis should suggest the possibility of infection. Investigation by computed tomographic (CT) scan may reveal an aneurysm at an atypical site and/or a vascular mass contiguous with the aorta. There may be loss of tissue planes in the periaortic tissues. Angiogram shows an aneurysm which is often saccular and eccentric with normal proximal and distal vessels.

The bacteria involved may include salmonellae, staphylococci or anaerobic bacteria. The prognosis is said to be worst in patients with Gram-negative infection.

Surgical treatment is required urgently because early rupture is a frequent complication. The surgical management remains controversial, with the basic division being between those who place an intra-abdominal synthetic graft and those who use extra-anatomical bypass for reconstruction. The alternative techniques are described on page 228.

PRIMARY AORTOENTERIC FISTULA

This refers to a fistula developing in patients who have not had previous aortic surgery. This is a rare event. Underlying causes include aortic aneurysm, which is the most common cause, infection of the aorta (see above), adjacent tumour and peptic ulcer. In 80% of cases the fistula involves the duodenum. The clinical features and management are as described for secondary fistula (see p. 228). The absence of scarring and adhesions may make the approach to the lesion easier than in the more common secondary fistula.

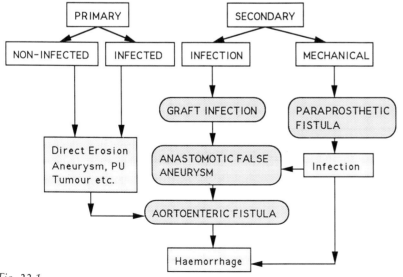

Fig. 22.1
Classification of infection.

INFECTED AORTIC GRAFT

This is the most dangerous site for a graft infection because of the risks of rupture into either the retroperitoneal space or the adjacent bowel, and because of the technical difficulties of removing and replacing an infected graft.

This condition may be difficult to diagnose because the initial symptoms are non-specific. The condition should be suspected in any patient with unexplained fever or other evidence of deep sepsis following aortic surgery. Virtually all of these patients have received antibiotic therapy and the acute signs of infection may be suppressed. Persistence or recurrence of back pain is common. Occlusion of one limb of an aortobifemoral graft or septic emboli to the lower limbs should raise the suspicion of graft infection.

CT scanning is the major diagnostic test and provides better resolution than ultrasound. CT scanning will demonstrate oedema, a loss of definition of tissue planes and sometimes gas in the tissues around the graft. There may also be a collection of fluid around the graft, but, especially early postoperatively, it may be difficult to determine if this is abnormal. A sample of this fluid may be aspirated under CT control for bacteriological analysis. CT scan may reveal alternative causes for the patient's symptoms not related to the arterial graft. Radionuclide scans are not sufficiently specific to allow confident diagnosis.

It is sometimes possible to suppress and probably cure some of these patients with aggressive and prolonged antibiotic therapy. If signs of sepsis persist or if signs of gastrointestinal haemorrhage occur, operation should be undertaken and the graft removed as described below.

FALSE ANEURYSM—NON INFECTED

Published evidence suggests that these lesions are rare, occurring in 1–6% of patients following aortic grafting. However, there are recent reports which suggest that they may be more common than are currently recognized. Edwards et al (1992) found aneurysms > 4 cm diameter in 8% of patients submitted to ultrasound examination.

It may present as a recurrence of an aneurysmal mass in the abdomen or with signs of leakage of blood from the aorta. The aetiology is failure of the anastomosis either from breaking of the suture or from the wall of the aorta giving way. Risk factors for false aneurysm such as postoperative sepsis, steroid therapy, urgent operation and renal failure will be present in about half the patients. This lesion may be indistinguishable from a new aneurysm forming in the aorta above the graft.

When the aneurysm presents before rupture, CT scanning and angiography should be performed to delineate the lesion and the relationship to it of the renal vessels. Asymptomatic lesions detected by screening examination may be treated conservatively if they are small and if there are no signs of progressive enlargement. The evidence of Edwards et al (1992) suggests that most of these will remain asymptomatic, at least in the short term.

SECONDARY AORTOENTERIC FISTULA

Incidence
The true incidence is unknown. The best estimates suggest that it occurs in about 1% of patients following repair of an abdominal aortic aneurysm.

Pathogenesis
There are two major explanations for the development of this complication. The 'mechanical' theory is that the graft, in the region of the proximal anastomosis, erodes into the duodenum which is fixed by scar tissue. Local infection occurs and the anastomosis fails, resulting in bleeding from the aorta into the duodenum. Support for this explanation comes from the occasional finding of erosion of the duodenal wall in contact with the mid portion of the graft, away from the anastomosis. Such a finding on endoscopy usually results in an urgent call to the vascular surgeon. This is called a paraprosthetic 'fistula' (see definitions above).

The 'infection' theory postulates that a false aneurysm occurs as a result of infection in the proximal anastomosis. This aneurysm ruptures into the adjacent duodenum. Thus in these cases, infection is the major aetiological factor and this has important implications for the method of treatment used. Graft infection is often detected following a secondary intervention for occlusion of one limb of an aortobifemoral graft. It is suggested that the intervention has caused the infection. An alternative explanation, which we favour, is that the occlusion was the presenting feature of an infected graft.

Clinical features
The commonest presentation (in about two-thirds of patients) is with a major gastrointestinal haemorrhage usually, but not always, with haematemesis. In about 25% of patients the bleeding will be chronic or intermittent and this should suggest the presence of a paraprosthetic fistula. Sometimes there have not been significant preceding symptoms but in many cases there will have been features suggesting a graft infection (see above). There is a past history of aortic surgery months to years previously. (About 10% present within the first month after surgery.)

The combination of a history of aortic surgery, sepsis and gastrointestinal haemorrhage indicates the presence of an aortoduodenal fistula until another diagnosis is proven.

Gastroduodenal endoscopy is the most valuable method of diagnosis. The endoscope must be passed as far into the duodenum as possible. The probability of aortoenteric fistula is heightened if gastroduodenal endoscopy does not reveal a source for the haemorrhage or if the haemorrhage is seen to be distal to the second part of the duodenum. A fistula may be seen as an ulcer or area of oedema and inflammation in the third part of the duodenum, or in some cases the graft may be seen. It must be remembered that the presence of an ulcer in the first part of the duodenum does not exclude the presence of an aortoenteric fistula. CT scanning may reveal evidence of a perigraft infection (see above) or a false aneurysm. As mentioned previously, there is commonly a small 'warning' haemorrhage before the major rupture. There are not usually any previous symptoms to suggest the presence of peptic ulcer, although this condition is more common in patients with aortic disease.

PARAPROSTHETIC 'FISTULA'

As indicated in the figure, this is one of the manifestations of graft infection and should be anticipated in any patient with an aortic graft infection. Patients with this condition are more septic than patients with infected grafts in whom the duodenum is intact. The condition may be difficult to diagnose because the imaging techniques usually used are insensitive in diagnosing the defect in the bowel. Chronic or intermittent gastrointestinal blood loss occurs in about 25% of cases.

MANAGEMENT OF AORTIC INFECTION AND AORTOENTERIC FISTULA

These are major complications, with a significant risk to the life of the patient.

Preoperative care
Careful preparation of the patient is mandatory:

1.   Angiography will be performed to provide information about the state of all anastomoses and of arteries which may be used for new distal anastomoses. Angiography may not be possible in cases of severe haemorrhage.
2.   There must be rigorous efforts to identify the infecting organisms and to treat them with appropriate antibiotics for 7–10 days preoperatively if possible.
3.   Chronically septic patients may benefit from a period of hyperalimentation.

Blood loss may be considerable and supracoeliac clamping will be necessary in most cases. A Swan–Ganz catheter should be inserted and early in the procedure an infusion of mannitol commenced. The anaesthetist should be warned that urgent supracoeliac clamping may be necessary and should be prepared to manage rapid blood loss and/or the effects of high clamping of the aorta.

A patient with active bleeding from an aortoenteric fistula should be transferred to the operating theatre as soon as possible and prepared as a patient with a ruptured abdominal aortic aneurysm.

Operation
A number of the steps in these operations have been described in previous sections, to which reference is made in this section.

If it is planned to remove an aortobifemoral graft completely and if

there is no active haemorrhage occurring, both groins should be dissected before opening the abdomen. The anastomosis of the prosthesis to the femoral artery must be displayed. If the groin is infected further dissection of the outflow vessels should not be undertaken at this stage for fear of infecting the planned new distal anastomosis.

The abdomen should be opened through the previous incision. After dividing any adhesions, the area of the aorta is approached.

False aneurysm or fistula at proximal anastomosis
The anastomosis should not be approached directly during the initial dissection unless the preoperative studies have shown that there is a substantial length (2–3 cm) of aorta available below the renal arteries. It will be unusual to find these conditions in patients who have had a previous repair of an abdominal aortic aneurysm. However, in patients who have had an aortobifemoral bypass with an end-to-side aortic anastomosis it is usually possible to dissect and control the infrarenal aorta.

An elective approach should be made to the supracoeliac aorta as described on page 144. When this has been done, preparations should be made to apply a clamp to this area immediately should the need arise.

The distal common iliac arteries should be dissected as described on page 135. Adhesions may make the search for the ureters difficult.

Only then should the proximal anastomosis be approached directly. The objective is to delay as long as possible the inadvertent opening of the aneurysm. The principles of the exposure are similar to those for other secondary procedures. The approach should start in tissue which has not been dissected previously. In areas like the origin of the renal arteries, this is easier said than done. However, a plane should be sought in relatively undisturbed tissues. This may be high up on the anterior aspect of the aorta, in the region of the superior mesenteric artery or on the left side below the renal artery. The left renal vein may be difficult to identify and dissect because of fibrosis. The aim is to identify and dissect both renal arteries first and then dissect the region of the neck of the aneurysm. The lower part of the graft can be displayed by incising the wall of the original aneurysm wrapped around the graft. There is a clear plane of cleavage between the two (see arrow in Fig. 22.2).

If the dissection is completed before opening the aneurysm, it may be possible to place an infrarenal clamp. These are the ideal circumstances. If this is not possible, the supracoeliac clamp and a clamp distally on the graft should be applied. The aneurysm cavity may be approached directly or by incising the prosthesis in its upper part until the region of the anastomosis has been reached. Excessive back-bleeding from the visceral arteries can be controlled by intraluminal balloon catheters.

The succeeding steps depend on the particular condition being treated.

Anastomotic false aneurysm—non infected. Thrombus is removed and redundant false aneurysm wall excised. The prosthesis is completely separated from the aorta at the proximal anastomosis. A new piece of prosthesis of appropriate diameter is sutured end to end to the aorta. There is usually room to make this anastomosis below the renal arteries but the techniques described on pages 156—158 may need to be used. When this anastomosis is complete, the supracoeliac clamp is removed and a clamp placed across the graft. The graft

is cut to an appropriate length and anastomosed end to end to the original graft. Care must be taken to cover the prosthesis completely so that the duodenum is separated by a layer of living tissue. The wall of the aneurysm or omentum can be used. To obtain additional length of tissue, the omentum may be mobilized on a pedicle which includes the right gastroepiploic vessels.

Infected false aneurysm. The management of this condition is controversial. The conventional teaching is that all the

graft must be removed and repair performed using autogenous tissues or extra-anatomical techniques for reconstruction. Autogenous repairs are not applicable to patients who have had surgery for abdominal aortic aneurysm. The alternative is to close the aortic stump and perform extra-anatomical reconstruction such as axillobifemoral bypass, but there is no way of closing the aortic stump which is guaranteed not to burst at some later time.

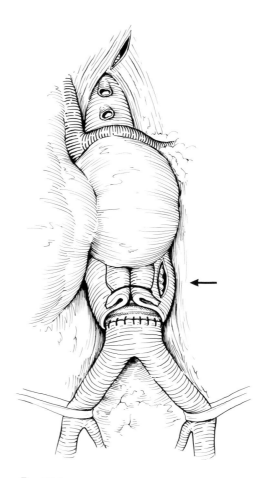

Fig. 22.2
Dissection of false aneurysm at upper anastomosis.

There have been several reports of local repair or the insertion of a new prosthesis. This cuts across the general principle in surgery that if there is a foreign body in an infected field, the infection will not resolve until the foreign material has been removed. Successful outcomes have been reported in situations where there is no alternative to local reconstruction such as the suprarenal aorta and where alternative approaches are available. Both approaches will be described.

1. *Conventional.* Staged repair may be possible. The axillofemoral bypass can be placed some days before removing the graft and this approach may have a lower mortality. The rate of amputation is increased if restoration of the circulation distally is delayed. If the two stages are to be performed under the same anaesthetic, the reconstruction is performed before removing the infected graft, provided the condition of the patient allows.

The aorta is prepared as described above. After application of clamps the previous graft is excised. Infected graft is not firmly attached to the surrounding tissues. However, in most cases the distal limbs of an aortobifemoral graft will not be infected and will be firmly invested by fibrous tissue. Removal of these parts may be difficult and bloody and great care must be taken to identify and protect the ureters. One technique which may assist is to pass a Bakes dilator up from the groin in the lumen of the graft. The dilator is sutured to the cut iliac limb of the graft. As the dilator is withdrawn, the graft is inverted and pulled away from the surrounding tissue. An alarming amount of force may be required to apply this method and the surgeon may desist because of lack of progress.

Infected and damaged tissue in the region of the aorta is excised and the aortic wall trimmed until healthy tissue is obtained. This may result in the need to reimplant one or both renal arteries. The end of the aorta is closed. Interrupted sutures placed as deeply as possible are used (Fig. 22.3). They must be tied very carefully so that they are not so tight that they will tear out of the aorta when the clamp is released. It may be very difficult to complete this suture line satisfactorily. The suture line is covered with omentum. Innovative techniques such as serosal patching and use of the anterior spinal ligament to cover the aortic suture line have been advocated but there is no evidence that they reduce the incidence of disruption of the aortic stump. The graft is removed from the lower anastomosis and the lower end of the aorta oversewn.

2. *In situ repair.* The operation proceeds as described above until the graft has been removed and the damaged tissue excised. A length of PTFE 12 mm in diameter is cut at an angle of about 45° (Fig. 22.4). This is sutured to the aorta so that the body of the prosthesis lies to the left. When the anastomosis is complete, the graft is passed deep to the left colonic mesentery (Fig. 22.5) into the left paracolic gutter and lateral to the colon to pass beneath the inguinal ligament. That part of the graft between the aorta and the mesocolon is covered with omentum. The abdomen is closed and the prosthesis anastomosed to the side of the common femoral artery. The reconstruction is completed by performing a femoral crossover graft (Fig. 22.6).

Aortoenteric fistula
The surgical approach should be as described above. If there is active haemorrhage the supracoeliac clamp should be applied as quickly as possible. The lower part of the prosthesis is exposed through the wall of the former aneurysm (Fig. 22.2) and clamped.

In most cases there are no obvious signs of infection and the duodenum is densely adherent to the region of the proximal anastomosis. Sometimes there will be an abscess cavity between the two. In the more common case, a scalpel is used to separate the duodenum from the aorta. Leakage of duodenal content is controlled by the application of non-crushing clamps.

The next steps will depend on the size of the hole in the aortic anastomosis and the degree of infection present. The conventional method is to assume that the graft is infected, excise it all and carry out an axillobifemoral bypass. There will inevitably be contamination with organisms from the duodenum but invasive infection is uncommon. Therefore, it is argued that local repair, with appropriate antibiotic cover, is a reasonable and safe procedure. If the defect in the anastomosis is small it may be repaired directly. More commonly, the anastomosis is taken down completely and a new piece of prosthetic material anastomosed to the aorta at the site of the previous anastomosis. Distally, an end-to-end anastomosis is performed between the new and original prostheses. The prosthesis is covered with omentum.

The duodenum is mobilized so that the defect in it can be closed transversely or obliquely to avoid narrowing. A drain should be placed close to the duodenal suture line. If the defect in the duodenum is large, a feeding jejunostomy may be placed to provide a route for enteral nutrition. This not only protects the duodenal anastomosis but allows early feeding which may be advantageous in patients who have been chronically septic.

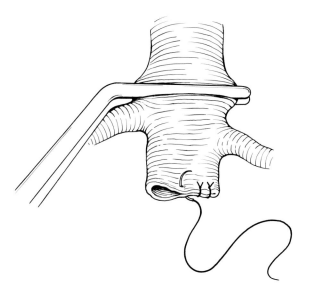

Fig. 22.3
Closure of aortic stump. Clamps on renal arteries not shown.

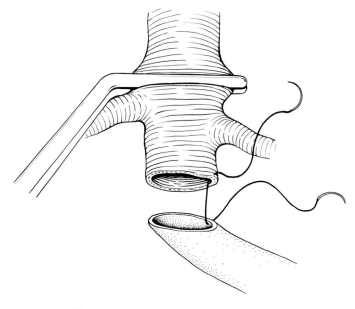

Fig. 22.4
Beginning of anastomosis between aorta and PTFE.

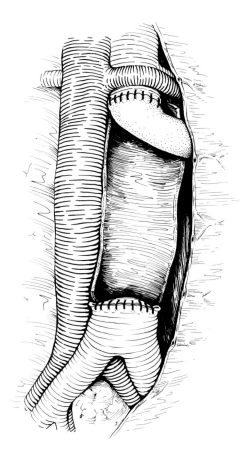

Fig. 22.5
Ccmpleted anastomosis with PTFE passing beneath mesocolon.

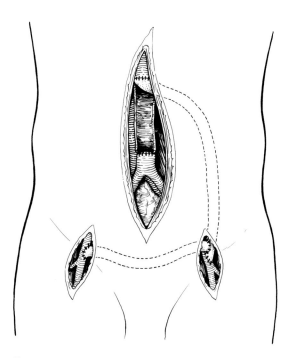

Fig. 22.6
Anatomy of completed reconstruction.

Paraprosthetic 'fistula'
The duodenum is mobilized from the prosthesis and closed as described. If there is minimal evidence of infection, the prosthesis may be covered with omentum and left in place. If the body of the graft is infected but the anastomoses intact and well incorporated in fibrous tissue, clamps may be applied to the graft without the need for major proximal and distal dissection. The intermediate segment is excised and a new prosthesis inserted and anastomosed end to end to the remaining ends of the original graft. If the whole length of the graft is infected, it should be treated as described above.

Postoperative care

In all cases where an infected graft has been encountered, the patient should receive prolonged antibiotic therapy in the postoperative period. There should be a high index of suspicion for recurrent infection.

Results

Few centres have a large experience of treating these patients and many series report a high mortality. Reilly et al (1987) have reported a large experience with a mortality for aortoenteric fistula of 36% and 17% with infection but no fistula. The amputation rate was 28% for patients with infected aortofemoral grafts. Recurrent or persistent infection occurred in 27%.

REFERENCES

Edwards J M, Teefey S A, Zierler R E, Kohler T R 1992 Abdominal aortic pseudoaneurysms after aortic bypass grafting. Journal of Vascular Surgery 15: 344–353
Reilly L M, Stoney R J, Goldstone J, Ehrenfeld W K 1987 Improved management of aortic graft infection: the influence of operation sequence and staging. Journal of Vascular Surgery 5: 421–431

Chapter 23

Infection and false aneurysm in other sites

Introduction

These complications may occur at any arterial suture line. The common femoral artery is overwhelmingly the most common location. Aneurysm at this site will be described in detail. The principles can be applied at other sites.

1. ANASTOMOTIC NON-INFECTED ANEURYSM

Approximately 80% of anastomotic aneurysms occur in the groin. The most common previous procedure is aortofemoral bypass grafting. The incidence is between 0.5% and 4%. About 50% of these aneurysms appear within 3–4 years of the initial operation but they may occur at any time following operation. The incidence of femoral anastomotic aneurysms following femorodistal bypass surgery is < 1%.

PATHOGENESIS

This has been described most convincingly by Courbier & Aboukhater (1988). Their account focuses on the effect that the inguinal ligament has on a prosthetic graft passing beneath it. Tethering of the graft to the ligament produces forces which tend to tear the apex of the anastomosis from the artery on extension of the hip. Thus it is common to find that the proximal part of the anastomosis is intact but the prosthesis has pulled away from the distal end. Sometimes the suture is broken; on other occasions the suture is intact but has pulled through the wall of the artery. Other factors which have been reported to be important include weakening of the wall of the artery by endarterectomy or by the sutures and stresses occurring because of the different compliance between the artery and prosthesis.

A history of local wound complications is more common in patients with false aneurysm. As a consequence attention has turned to the possibility of infection as the cause. Despite the absence of local or systemic features of infection, bacteria of normally low pathogenicity can be isolated in a proportion of cases. It is generally considered that these lesions should be considered infected until proven otherwise. Antibiotic prophylaxis is essential and specimens of tissue and graft should be sent for culture, particularly seeking *Staphylococcus epidermidis*.

There is a small but definite incidence of recurrent anastomotic aneurysm but this is hardly surprising given the local factors which are presumed to be involved in the aetiology. The recurrence rate following conventional local repair does not suggest that these techniques should be abandoned in favour of the more radical methods for treating infected grafts.

CLINICAL FEATURES

The patient usually complains of a lump in one groin several years following aortofemoral bypass. The natural history is of gradual expansion of the lump until rupture occurs. This is indicated by the sudden onset of pain and rapid enlargement of the mass with haemorrhage into the subcutaneous tissues. Necrosis of the skin due to this haemorrhage is a sign that emergency repair should be undertaken.

DIAGNOSTIC TESTS

Angiography has been the commonest method for determining the anatomy of these lesions (Fig. 23.1). However, adequate information can be obtained non-invasively by means of duplex ultrasound which can demonstrate the site and size of the aneurysm and the state of the superficial and, more importantly, the profunda femoris arteries. It must be remembered that angiography only demonstrates the lumen, not the external diameter of the aneurysm.

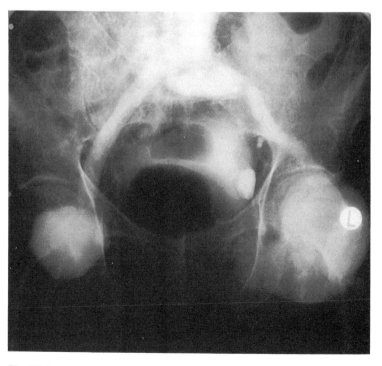

Fig. 23.1
Angiogram of bilateral femoral anastomotic aneurysms.

Prophylactic antibiotics should be given because prosthetic material will be inserted. Part of the thrombus from the aneurysm should be sent for culture.

INDICATIONS FOR OPERATION

An aneurysm which is greater than 2.5 cm in diameter or which is enlarging or the source of emboli should be repaired.

OPERATION

Preparation
The potential operation field includes the skin from the umbilicus to the knee. This area should be prepared and draped. A sterile towel which can be removed easily is placed over the lower abdomen.

Incision
The aim is to obtain control of the vessels above and below the site of the disruption. In large or ruptured aneurysms, the vessels are first controlled in the iliac fossa. This allows the inflow to be occluded quickly should the aneurysm be opened inadvertently during the dissection. In small aneurysms this may not be necessary and the dissection at the level of the inguinal ligament should precede dissection of the distal vessels.

To control the iliac vessels an oblique incision is made in the iliac fossa as in the approach to an appendicectomy (Fig. 23.2). The muscle layers can be split or the deeper layers divided if necessary to provide adequate exposure. The graft is approached extraperitoneally and mobilized sufficiently to allow a clamp to be placed across it. The position of the ureter may have been distorted by previous dissection and care must be taken not to damage it (Fig. 23.3).

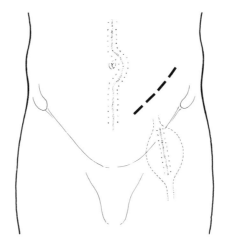

Fig. 23.2
Abdominal incision to control external iliac artery.

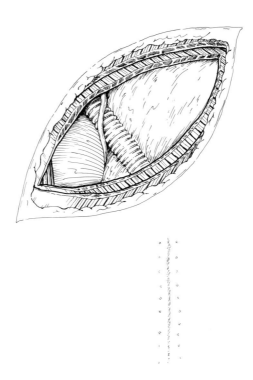

Fig. 23.3
Graft and ureter displayed—seen from left side.

The lower part of the original femoral incision is opened and extended distally for 2–4 cm (Fig. 23.4). This allows the superficial femoral artery to be approached in an area away from the aneurysm. The superficial femoral artery is encircled at a convenient point distal to the aneurysm. The dissection then proceeds proximally along the front and sides of the superficial femoral artery (Fig. 23.5). The aneurysm is usually well encapsulated and the larger part of the lumen occupied with solid thrombus. The aneurysm can be lifted forwards to allow the dissection to approach the origin of the profunda femoris artery. Sharp dissection is preferred as in all re-do surgery. An assistant holds the aneurysm while the surgeon stretches the tissues around the artery and cuts as close as possible to the vessel. With patience, a plane close to the artery can be found. The dissection may often be carried along the sides of the femoral vessels and the aneurysm as shown in Figure 23.6. It is good if the profunda femoris artery can be identified and dissected but this step is not essential, as long as there has been sufficient dissection along the vessels to allow application of a clamp across both the superficial femoral artery and the profunda femoris artery.

The next step is to dissect the graft as it passes beneath the inguinal ligament. The proximal part of the old femoral incision is reopened and extended proximally until it is certain that it is over the inguinal ligament.

The proximal part of the wound is deepened until fibres of the external oblique muscle are identified. These are followed distally until the inguinal ligament is seen (Fig. 23.7). The lower border of the inguinal ligament is defined by sharp dissection as far as possible (2–3 cm) on each side of the graft. The graft is approached by deepening this incision on each side of the aneurysm, retracting it as necessary.

If the femoral vein is identified medially, it is a good indication of the depth of the common femoral artery. The graft is approached by retracting the inguinal ligament and deepening the dissection at its distal edge (Fig. 23.8). This dissection is inclined proximally and the graft can be identified. Using sharp dissection and keeping as close to the graft as possible, the anterior and lateral aspects of the prosthesis are dissected sufficiently to allow application of a clamp. It may be possible to separately dissect the common femoral artery but this is not an essential step.

It should now be possible to apply clamps to the prosthesis as it emerges from beneath the inguinal ligament and to the superficial femoral artery and profunda femoris artery. The clamp is applied to the profunda femoris artery as shown in Figure 23.9. As pointed out above, this can be done without the need to formally dissect the profunda femoris artery.

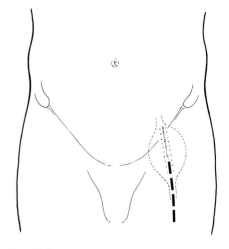

Fig. 23.4
Incision extending distal to old wound.

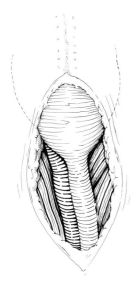

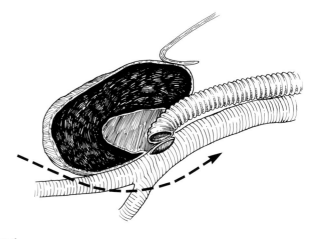

Fig. 23.6
Sagittal section through aneurysm showing plane of dissection from distal to proximal.

Fig. 23.5
Control of superficial femoral artery below aneurysm.

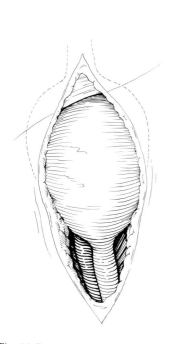

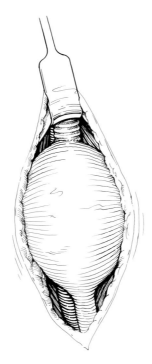

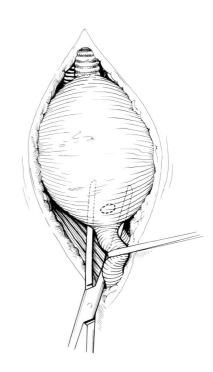

Fig. 23.7
Dissection of proximal aneurysm: inguinal ligament overlying aneurysm.

Fig. 23.8
Graft entering aneurysm.

Fig. 23.9
Positioning of clamp to control profunda femoris artery.

The aneurysm is incised and the laminated thrombus removed. The site of the disruption of the anastomosis can be seen as shown in Figure 23.10. Bleeding may occur from the femoral artery if the external iliac artery is patent or from the deep circumflex iliac and the deep epigastric arteries which arise as the external iliac artery passes beneath the inguinal ligament (see Fig. 20.1). This bleeding may be controlled by a balloon catheter in the common femoral artery (Fig. 23.11). Further dissection of the prosthesis and common femoral artery may be undertaken in the lumen of the aneurysm.

The region of the anastomosis is inspected. In the example illustrated (Fig. 23.10), the graft had pulled away from the artery and the suture had broken. Given the presumed aetiology of these lesions, it is not appropriate to perform a direct repair of the suture line because this will only reinstate the conditions which led to the formation of the aneurysm. Additional length of graft is needed and there is evidence that recurrence is less frequent when an interposition graft is used (Ernst et al 1988).

The prosthesis is completely separated from the artery and lifted forwards as far as possible. This allows good exposure of the common femoral artery, which can be dissected and clamped. The intimal lining of the artery can be seen clearly. The wall of the aneurysm should be cut away from the artery so that sutures can be placed in the wall of the artery and not in the fibrous tissue forming the wall of the aneurysm. This is an important principle because suturing to fibrous tissue will predispose to recurrence. A length of prosthetic material is selected. This should be of the same diameter as the original prosthesis. One end is cut obliquely to match the size of the defect in the common femoral artery.

This end is sutured to the defect in the artery. A variety of techniques may be used. In the illustration (Fig. 23.12), the anastomosis has started at the proximal end and the side away from the surgeon is being sutured from within the lumen of the artery. It is important to ensure that adequate bites of the wall of the artery are taken. In some cases the anastomosis may be performed end to end to the common orifices of the superficial femoral artery and the profunda femoris artery as illustrated in Figure 20.3. This would be performed if the common femoral artery is extensively damaged or of poor quality.

When the anastomosis between new prosthesis and common femoral artery has been completed, the old prosthesis is cut transversely and sutured end to end to the new prosthesis (Fig. 23.13).

The clamps are removed and blood flow restored to the leg. Redundant tissue from the wall of the false aneurysm should be cut away. The wound is closed in the usual manner.

RESULTS

The results of surgery are good, with low mortality and amputation rates. However, the risks are significantly higher for those requiring emergency surgery. The prognosis is that of the underlying atherosclerosis.

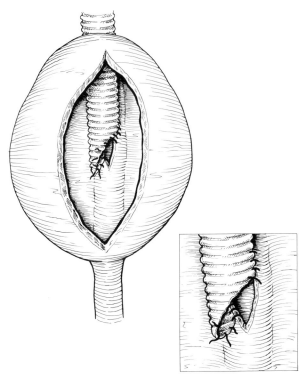

Fig. 23.10
Anatomy of lesion: partial disruption of anastomosis.

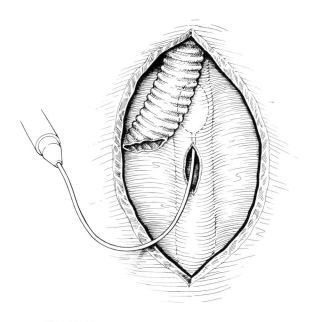

Fig. 23.11
Control of common femoral artery by balloon catheter.

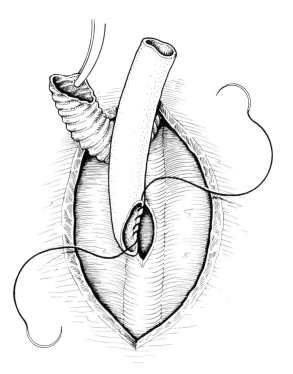

Fig. 23.12
Suture of new graft to defect in common femoral artery.

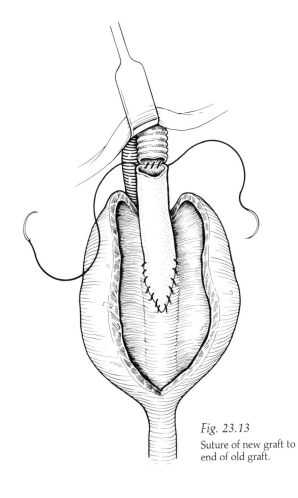

Fig. 23.13
Suture of new graft to
end of old graft.

2. INFECTED FALSE ° ANEURYSM

Infection in an arterial prosthesis is one of the most feared complications of arterial surgery because the infected graft carries a threat to both life and limb. Fortunately the complication is rare (1–2% of arterial reconstructions) but when it occurs there may be major problems in determining and carrying out appropriate management. Infection may occur at any time after a vascular operation.

The principles of management are to:

1. Control haemorrhage.
2. Drain the infection.
3. Restore the distal circulation.

Even if this is achieved satisfactorily, there may be delayed problems from recurrent infection.

The commonest site of infection in an arterial anastomosis is the groin. This is presumably because of the difficulties of removing all bacteria from the skin in this area and of maintaining aseptic technique. About half the patients present with an intact anastomosis and half with false aneurysm. The following description gives a detailed account of the management of infection in the groin. The principles described are applicable to other sites. Infection in an aortic prosthesis has been described on page 228.

PATHOGENESIS

Superficial infections and minor wound breakdown are common in procedures to revascularize the lower limb. They may not be serious in themselves but they carry a higher risk of infection of the arterial anastomoses beneath. There are three ways in which infection may develop:

1. Direct spread from wound infection. This results in a cellulitis involving the region of the anastomosis. Suppuration may follow. These infections present within days to weeks after surgery.

2. Late infection with organisms of low pathogenicity whose growth has been potentiated by the presence of a foreign body, namely the prosthetic graft. The common organism is *Staphylococcus epidermidis*. This topic has been discussed under the heading of Anastomotic false aneurysm on page 236. Many of these cases represent infection which has occurred at the time of the primary operation and which has been suppressed by perioperative administration of antibiotics.

3. Late infection as a consequence of bacteraemia. These infections are analogous to bacterial endocarditis developing on prosthetic heart valves. For this reason a patient with a prosthetic arterial graft must be given prophylactic antibiotics in the same way as a patient at risk of bacterial endocarditis.

Infection results in disruption of the wall of the vessel (artery or vein graft). This disruption occurs at or close to the anastomosis. With disruption of the wall, haemorrhage occurs. This may be contained, resulting in a false aneurysm. However, the haemorrhage seldom remains localized and free rupture soon occurs. The rate of progression is more rapid in the presence of infection than in non-infected false aneurysm.

CLINICAL FEATURES

The severity of the systemic symptoms vary from a severe toxic illness to no systemic upset. In the acute infections there will be signs of cellulitis extending beyond the margins of the wound. There may be the discharge of pus from the wound resulting in a sinus which persists. Before major haemorrhage occurs there is often one or more small haemorrhages from the wound. This is a sign which should not be overlooked. Free rupture is a dramatic event and unless the attending staff act appropriately death from exsanguination may occur.

PREOPERATIVE PREPARATION

It is preferable to operate on these patients before haemorrhage occurs. Identification of the infecting organisms and their sensitivities to antibiotics is essential. There must be adequate supplies of blood available to meet the anticipated need for transfusion.

OPERATION

Control of haemorrhage

If haemorrhage occurs, the patient will usually be transferred to the operating theatre, with an attendant applying pressure constantly to the groin. This should provide adequate, if temporary, control of the bleeding and allow the circulating blood volume to be restored before proceeding. When the patient has been anaesthetized, the skin is prepared in a wide area, leaving until last the area from which the haemorrhage is coming. The pressure is released, the area prepared and temporary drapes applied if bleeding recurs.

The method used to control the haemorrhage will depend on the amount of bleeding and the time since the previous operation. If the operation has been recent, the tissue planes will be found easily and it will be possible to obtain precise control of the bleeding site. In these cases, the wound is opened directly and the vessels controlled, first with digital pressure and then with clamps. If these conditions are unlikely to be found, control of the graft and/or external iliac artery should be obtained as described on page 237. Distal control may be obtained by the insertion of balloon catheters (see p. 241).

Drainage of infection

Specimens should be taken for bacteriological analysis. The patient should receive large doses of antibiotics to cover the most common pathogens (*Staphylococcus aureus* and *S. epidermidis*, coliforms and anaerobic Bacteroides species). Areas of suppuration should be drained and dead tissue excised.

Reconstruction

The general principle is that all foreign material should be removed and a repair performed using autogenous tissues. If it is essential to use prosthetic material, the graft should be placed in an uninfected bed and anastomosed to uninfected artery. The precise technique used depends on the previous surgery.

Previous proximal reconstruction

The proximal extent of the infection must be determined. Commonly the infection involves one limb of an aortobifemoral graft, with the aortic anastomosis and the opposite limb uninvolved.

The graft is exposed through the iliac fossa (Figures 22.2 and 22.3). The signs of infection involving the graft at this level are the presence of pus or cellulitis and the degree of incorporation of the graft. In infected prosthetic grafts, the prosthesis lies loosely in the connective tissue sheath and the graft can be easily lifted from its bed. Non-infected grafts are adherent to the surrounding tissues and can only be removed by sharp dissection. If the graft is not infected at this level it is clamped and transected.

The distal segment is withdrawn through the groin wound. Care should be taken to avoid damaging the ureter during this procedure.

A new piece of similar prosthesis is anastomosed end to end to the proximal cut end of the graft. There are several possible routes to the distal anastomosis, which will commonly be to the superficial femoral artery in mid-thigh. The easiest technique is to pass a long, curved forceps via the iliac fossa and beneath the lateral end of the inguinal ligament (if possible, avoiding the lateral cutaneous nerve of the thigh). The forceps are passed deep to the origin of the sartorius muscle and the tip exposed through a short incision through skin, subcutaneous tissue and fascia lata below and medial to the anterior superior iliac spine. The tips of a second, similar forceps are grasped in the jaws of the first forceps, which is then withdrawn into the abdomen. The prosthesis is grasped by the forceps passed from below and drawn into the thigh (Fig. 23.14). A similar incision is made 15–20 cm distally in the thigh and the graft placed in it in a similar manner. The tunnel is then carried medially to a convenient part of the mid-thigh where the superficial femoral artery is exposed. In this way, the new graft is placed in a clean field and the distal anastomosis performed end to side to healthy artery (Fig. 23.15).

Fig. 23.14
Passage of graft into thigh.

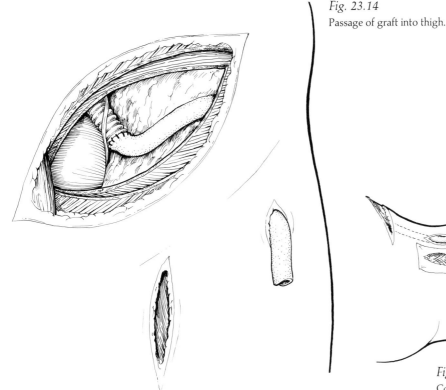

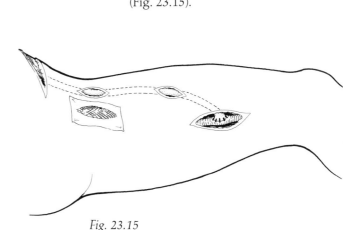

Fig. 23.15
Configuration of anastomosis to distal femoral artery.

If the graft in the iliac fossa is infected, the dissection should be carried up to the bifurcation of the graft. If it is incorporated at this level the graft is transected and oversewn. This is to avoid laying the new graft in the infected iliac fossa. Inflow to the limb is obtained from a crossover graft from the contralateral femoral region, the anastomosis being performed to either the prosthesis or the common femoral artery (Fig. 23.16).

If the infection extends above this level it should be treated as an infected aortic graft as described on page 228.

Obturator foramen
A more direct route to the thigh is via the obturator foramen. This can be felt as a depression in the floor of the pelvis, deep to the ramus of the pubis. Under direct vision, in a manner similar to that described above, the peritoneum and fascia over the obturator muscle can be incised, a forceps passed through the foramen (avoiding the obturator nerve) and the tip identified in the thigh. In this way, the new graft can be brought to the superficial femoral artery. Identification and passage of the obturator foramen is not as easy as is implied by the description above. The obturator nerve is very difficult to see. It may be possible to pass a tunneller from the thigh through the obturator membrane from below (Bell 1991).

Profunda femoris artery
If the superficial femoral artery is occluded, the distal anastomosis may be performed to the popliteal or profunda femoris artery. The latter is preferred because it will maintain the viability of the limb and a shorter prosthesis is needed.

Approach to the distal profunda femoris artery. It may be possible to approach the distal part of the profunda femoris artery without crossing the infected field related to the common femoral

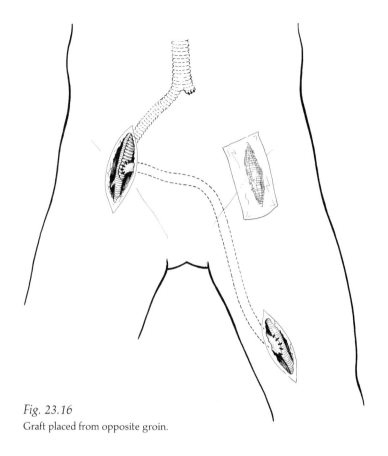

Fig. 23.16
Graft placed from opposite groin.

artery. An incision is made along the line of the sartorius muscle in the middle one-third of the thigh. The subsartorial canal is opened by displacing the muscle laterally and the superficial femoral artery mobilized (Fig. 23.17). Figure 23.18 shows a cross-section of the thigh, indicating the approach. The artery is displaced laterally and the lateral fibres of adductor longus muscle are incised parallel to the femur. The profunda femoris vessels are immediately deep to the muscle (Fig. 23.19). The artery is of sufficient calibre to receive a bypass graft.

Previous distal reconstruction
This represents infection in the proximal end of a femoropopliteal anastomosis. Inflow is obtained from the external iliac artery in the iliac fossa as described previously. A prosthesis of 6–8 mm PTFE or dacron may be used. The

prosthesis is placed in the thigh by one of the methods described above.

The distal anastomosis is performed to the previous graft in the mid-thigh. An end-to-end anastomosis is performed. If desired, a graft can be placed from the prosthesis to the distal profunda femoris artery.

Infected distal anastomosis following femorodistal surgery
The graft is transected at a convenient level through uninfected tissue. This is commonly around the level of the knee when the initial anastomosis has been to an artery below the knee. Every effort should be made to use autologous vein for the reconstruction, whether or not the initial procedure used autologous vein. Vein may be obtained from distally in the same limb, from the opposite limb or from the upper limb.

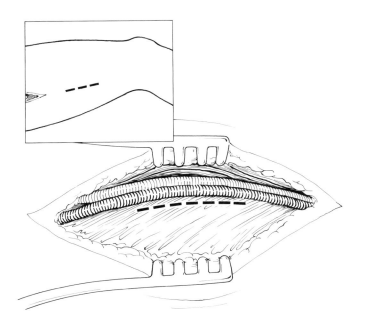

Fig. 23.17
Approach to distal profunda femoris artery.

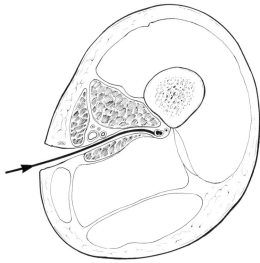

Fig. 23.18
Cross-section of approach to distal profunda femoris artery.

The distal anastomosis is fashioned to an appropriate artery in the calf in healthy tissue. The level should be as high as possible while avoiding the infected area. The tibioperoneal trunk or proximal posterior tibial artery are commonly used. If it is necessary to proceed more distally, the posterior tibial artery at the junction of the middle and lower third of the calf is the most accessible.

Infection in vein graft or vein in an infected field

The principle of replacing an infected graft with autologous material has been described. However, it should not be thought that autologous vein is immune to infection when placed in an infected field. Careful excision of dead tissue and a covering of healthy tissue are the best ways of reducing the chances of the vein becoming infected.

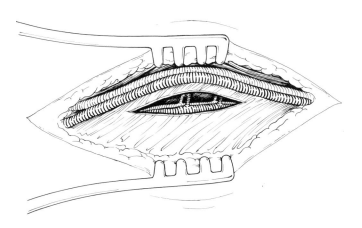

Fig. 23.19
Approach to distal profunda femoris artery—detail.

3. TRAUMATIC FALSE ANEURYSM

The topic of injuries to arteries is the subject of other texts and detailed consideration is beyond the scope of this account. Arteries to the limbs are most commonly injured. In geographical regions where knife and bullet wounds are uncommon, road trauma is the commonest cause. Penetrating trauma is the usual mechanism but closed injuries such as dislocation of the knee are a significant cause of morbidity.

In many referral centres the radiologist's catheter has replaced the knife or bullet as the commonest cause. When the femoral artery is used to provide access for endovascular procedures on the coronary arteries a sheath of external diameter 3 mm is commonly used. Given the size of this wound in the artery, it is surprising that serious problems occur as infrequently as they do.

The clinical features of arterial injury are haemorrhage and/or ischaemia. Note that ischaemia can occur in the absence of significant haemorrhage and the absence of ischaemia does not exclude the possibility of arterial injury. False aneurysm may result from partial division of an artery: either a puncture from a catheter or a side hole from knife or bullet. Another mechanism is distraction injury of the artery, when the inner layers of the arterial wall have been disrupted and the adventitia expands, producing a false aneurysm. These lesions may be seen at the origin of the brachiocephalic trunk or the subclavian artery. A bullet or knife passing through adjacent artery and vein may produce an arteriovenous fistula with or without false aneurysm.

In non-iatrogenic trauma angiography will be performed to define the site of injury. If there are multiple injuries to the patient this may be performed most conveniently in the operating theatre. A common scenario is a patient with fractures of the femur and tibia in the same limb. It may not be certain which of the fractures has caused the arterial injury. The femoral artery can be cannulated (after open exposure if necessary) and angiograms obtained. This procedure avoids the problems of transporting a severely injured patient to the radiology suite.

The principles of management of wounds of arteries are the same regardless of the particular artery injured (see p. 74 for an account of the management of rupture of the thoracic aorta). These principles are:

1.   Dissection of normal artery above and below the site of injury. The site of injury is approached along normal arteries. This is analogous to the approach to infected false aneurysms (see p. 228). If the false aneurysm sac is entered, clamps can be applied to control the haemorrhage while the site of injury is defined more clearly.
2.   Local repair is performed if the ends of the artery can be approximated without tension. Care must be taken to resect damaged artery and this usually means that an interposition graft must be inserted.
3.   In contaminated or infected wounds local repair with autogenous tissue may be performed. If it is necessary to use synthetic materials remote bypass should be performed as described in the management of infected false aneurysm (p. 242).
4.   Completion angiography should be performed to demonstrate the patency of the distal circulation. Two common sources of occlusion are a second injury distally and thromboembolism of the distal arterial tree.
5.   The timing of the arterial repair in

relation to fixation of fractures is controversial. My preference is to perform the arterial repair first and inspect it after the bones have been fixed. Others have described the use of arterial shunts while the bones are fixed. The worst situation is when the vascular surgeon is not called until after the bones have been fixed. This delay may result in irreversible ischaemic damage to muscle.

FALSE ANEURYSM OF THE FEMORAL ARTERY FOLLOWING CATHETERIZATION

Clinical features
The usual history is that there was extensive bruising in the groin following an endovascular procedure. As the peripheral bruising disappeared, the patient became conscious of a lump in the area of the puncture wound. This became more clearly defined as the swelling subsided. Smaller lumps (less than 2 cm in diameter) tend to disappear completely. Larger swellings may persist or expand. Rapid enlargement suggests infection and this is a very serious event. Infection occurs occasionally following coronary artery procedures but more commonly follows catheterization of the femoral vessels for haemodialysis in the intensive care unit.

Diagnostic tests
Duplex ultrasound is both diagnostic and therapeutic. Further angiography is unnecessary. Duplex scanning will reveal the size of the cavity containing liquid blood in relation to the size of the surrounding haematoma. The site of origin of the aneurysm from the common femoral artery can be determined. If the hole in the artery can be seen clearly and is less than 5 mm in diameter, it may be possible to occlude the aneurysm by applying pressure with the ultrasound probe over the hole and observing on the screen that flow in the aneurysm has ceased. After about

20 minutes the hole may be sealed and thus the examination may be therapeutic as well as diagnostic. There are now a number of reports of the use of this technique, which may succeed in obliterating the false aneurysm cavity in about 50% of cases. The chances of this manoeuvre being successful are reduced if the patient is receiving systemic anticoagulation.

Indications for operation
A mass greater than 2.5 cm in diameter which has persisted for several weeks or which is enlarging should be repaired. If there is an arteriovenous fistula present this should be repaired because spontaneous resolution is unlikely. Rapid enlargement or bleeding, in circumstances which suggest that infection may be present, should be dealt with as an emergency.

Preoperative care
A patient whose false aneurysm has occurred following coronary angiography may have severe, uncorrected coronary artery disease and therefore be at high risk of perioperative myocardial infarction. Sometimes it is preferable to repair the aneurysm at the time of coronary artery bypass grafting.

If infection is likely, blood cultures should be taken and antistaphylococcal therapy instituted.

Operation
In the absence of infection, the procedure is usually straightforward. The dissection is similar to that performed for false aneurysm at a femoral artery anastomosis as described earlier in this chapter. The incision is over the common femoral artery. Dissection in the subcutaneous tissue may be difficult because of the blood which has permeated the tissues. However, the planes of dissection around the arteries remain except in the area close to the site of injury. The relationship of the false aneurysm to the femoral artery is shown in Figure 23.20. The artery is exposed above and below the aneurysm (Figs 23.5 and 23.7) before the aneurysm is opened. It may not be possible to formally dissect the profunda femoris artery, which may need to be clamped as shown in Figure 23.9 or occluded with a balloon catheter after the artery has been opened.

After the application of the clamps the area of the aneurysm is approached from above and below. The haematoma is entered and the defect in the anterior wall of the common femoral artery displayed (Fig. 23.21).

The haematoma is removed and part of it sent for culture.

The defect in the artery is repaired. It is usually possible to close it directly with one or two sutures. These should be placed in the long axis of the artery to avoid narrowing the lumen. If the defect is too large to suture directly, it should be repaired using a small patch of autologous vein. This should be obtained from one of the tributaries of the long saphenous vein. The main trunk of the vein should be preserved.

If infection is present the reconstruction is much more difficult. Two approaches are possible.

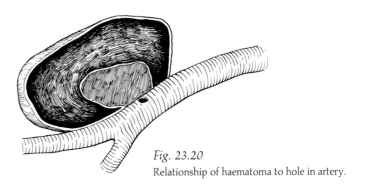

Fig. 23.20
Relationship of haematoma to hole in artery.

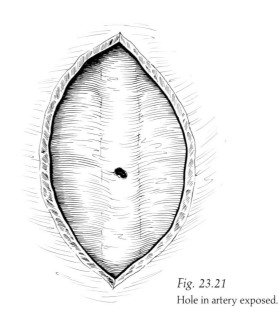

Fig. 23.21
Hole in artery exposed.

Conventional approach

In these patients the infected haematoma is removed. There is usually destruction of a major part of the wall of the common femoral artery. This means that some form of bypass needs to be performed.

Haematoma and infected arterial tissue are removed. This usually leaves the proximal part of the common femoral artery and may or may not preserve the bifurcation of the common femoral artery. The wound should be washed with antiseptic solution, the ends of the arteries oversewn, and the wounds closed.

Reconstruction is performed by placing a bypass graft from the external iliac artery, approached through a separate incision in the iliac fossa (Fig. 19.2), to the superficial femoral artery in the mid-thigh, away from the infected field (Fig. 23.15). If possible the distal profunda femoris artery should also be exposed (Fig. 23.18) and a graft placed to it. The graft may be routed as described above beneath the lateral part of the inguinal ligament or through the obturator foramen. The former route is easier. The graft used is usually PTFE 6–8 mm diameter.

Direct repair

In some cases it is appropriate to perform an arterial repair with prosthetic material in infected tissues (see discussion regarding aorta, p. 230). On several occasions we have treated false aneurysm in the groin following endovascular procedures by means of a PTFE inlay graft across the defect in the femoral artery. This simplifies the repair and may be an important factor in these critically ill patients. In all these situations there is a risk of secondary haemorrhage from infection and it is too early to say if the risk is excessive in these circumstances.

REFERENCES

Bell P R F 1991 Arterial surgery of the lower limb. Churchill Livingstone, Edinburgh, pp 77–85

Courbier R, Aboukhater R 1988 Progress in the treatment of anastomotic aneurysms. World Journal of Surgery 12: 742–749

Ernst C B, Elliott J P, Ryan C J et al 1988 Recurrent femoral anastomotic aneurysms: a 30 year experience. Annals of Surgery 208: 401–409

ANEURYSM OF BRANCHES OF THE THORACIC AND ABDOMINAL AORTA

Chapter 24

Aneurysm of branches of the thoracic aorta

1. BRACHIOCEPHALIC, SUBCLAVIAN AND AXILLARY ARTERY

These aneurysms are rare, comprising less than 1% of peripheral aneurysms. There are, however, several discrete patterns of aneurysms which can be recognized.

AETIOLOGY

Aneurysms of the brachiocephalic trunk and intrathoracic left subclavian artery may be degenerative and associated with other aneurysms in about 50% of cases. Aneurysms may also occur in patients with aortic dissection, syphilis, tuberculosis, Takayasu's arteritis and after trauma. Aneurysm may develop at the origin of a retro-oesophageal right subclavian artery from the aortic arch.

Aneurysms of the distal subclavian and proximal axillary artery are usually associated with a cervical rib.

True aneurysms of the axillary artery are very rare. The commonest cause of axillary aneurysm is damage to the artery from using crutches (see Neumayer et al 1992 for review). The pathology of these true aneurysms demonstrates fragmentation of elastic fibres in the wall and evidence of old haemorrhage into the wall. Macroscopically the aneurysm may be saccular or fusiform, associated with arteriomegaly. False aneurysms are more common. They result from blunt or penetrating trauma which may be iatrogenic. The presentation may be long after the trauma which initially might not be recognized as the cause.

CLINICAL FEATURES

Intrathoracic aneurysm may present as a consequence of pressure on adjacent structures, e.g. oesophagus or recurrent laryngeal nerve. Enlargement of an aneurysm may cause pain in the neck, chest or shoulder. Retrograde embolism of the carotid system may produce cerebral ischaemia.

Distal subclavian aneurysm associated with a cervical rib presents as abnormal pulsation in the neck or with symptoms of upper limb ischaemia.

The commonest cause of unilateral Raynaud's phenomenon is compression of the artery in the root of the neck.

The commonest presentation of axillary aneurysm is with a painless mass which is slowly enlarging. Symptoms of ischaemia of the hand and fingers may result from embolism of the thrombus from within the aneurysm. Direct pressure on adjacent nerves may cause pain. The aneurysm may be 6 cm or more in diameter when it presents. There have been few cases of rupture reported.

DIAGNOSIS

Clinical examination should allow a confident diagnosis of extrathoracic aneurysm. It is often difficult to differentiate between aneurysm and tortuosity of the arteries. Ultrasound will usually resolve the dilemma but angiography may be needed. Computed tomographic (CT) scanning will help detect significant intrathoracic lesions. Angiography will demonstrate the state of the proximal and distal arteries.

INDICATIONS FOR OPERATION

The rarity of these lesions makes it difficult to formulate general rules. Features suggesting progressive enlargement or rupture should be treated by operation. Operation should also be undertaken if there are symptoms of distal ischaemia or pressure on nerves. The first manifestation of a subclavian aneurysm may be limb-threatening ischaemia. In the presence of a cervical rib, any evidence of damage to the artery is an indication for removal of the rib. Small asymptomatic lesions may be treated expectantly.

OPERATION

Brachiocephalic or intrathoracic subclavian aneurysm

For brachiocephalic aneurysm a median sternotomy should be performed (Fig. 24.1). This may be extended into the neck along the anterior border of sternomastoid muscle if further exposure of the common carotid or subclavian artery is needed. The arteries are exposed after displacement of the thymus and retraction of the veins anterior to the arteries. A clamp is placed to partially occlude the aorta (Fig. 24.2). Further clamps are placed distal to the aneurysm. The aneurysm wall need not be excised completely if it is adherent to surrounding structures. A graft 10–12 mm in diameter is used to bridge the defect. In cases of extensive aneurysm a bifurcation graft may be used with the stem sutured to the aorta and the limbs sutured to the subclavian and common carotid arteries. In cases of trauma the wall of the aneurysm is the adventitial layers of the artery. The origin of the artery from the aorta should be oversewn and the proximal end of the graft placed to normal adjacent aorta. For aneurysm of the proximal left subclavian artery a left lateral thoracotomy should be undertaken.

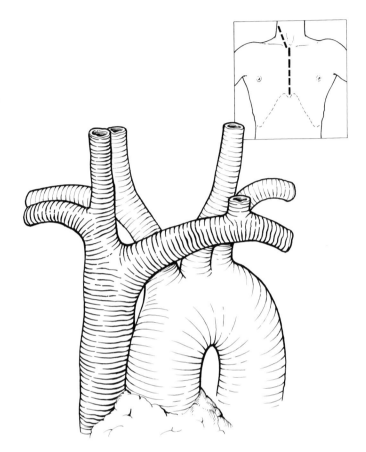

Fig. 24.1
Approach to brachiocephalic trunk.

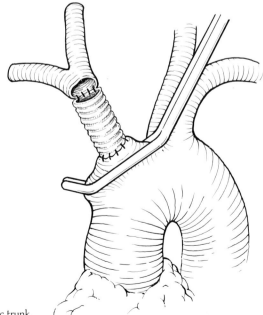

Fig. 24.2
Reconstruction of brachiocephalic trunk.

Supraclavicular exposure of the subclavian artery

This approach can be used to expose the subclavian and proximal axillary artery. On the right side the origin of the subclavian artery can be exposed and controlled. The head of the patient is placed on a head ring and the neck extended by placing a small sandbag beneath the shoulders. The head is turned to the opposite side and an incision made 1.5–2 cm above the clavicle. The medial end of the incision is the triangular space between the clavicular and sternal heads of the sternomastoid muscle and the incision is 5–6 cm long (Fig. 24.3). After division of the platysma muscle and the external jugular vein the cervical fascia is incised and the clavicular head of the sternomastoid muscle divided in the line of the incision. The posterior layer of the investing fascia is divided as far laterally as the inferior belly of the omohyoid muscle. The scalenus anterior muscle at the medial end of the wound is overlapped by the scalene fat pad, which may be mobilized superiorly. The subclavian vein may be found between the clavicle and the muscle and the subclavian artery felt emerging from the lateral edge of the muscle (Fig. 24.4). The scalenus anterior muscle and phrenic nerve lie behind the prevertebral fascia. The muscle is divided, taking care to avoid the phrenic nerve, which is usually at its medial edge at this level but which crosses the muscle anteriorly higher up. Division is best performed by lifting with dissecting forceps small bundles of muscle and cutting the bundles with scissors. As the deeper part of the muscle is approached the white tendinous fibres on the posterior aspect of the muscle can be seen. At this stage the lateral edge of the muscle may be divided, taking care not to injure the artery. Some advocate passing a dissector or forceps behind the tendon but this is not necessary and may be difficult. Injury to the artery is best avoided by lifting the tendinous fibres forward, away from the artery. Once the scalenus anterior muscle is divided, the whole length of the anterior aspect of the cervical subclavian artery can be exposed. The disposition of the branches is as shown in Figure 24.5. An encircling tape should be passed around the artery distal to the vertebral artery.

In patients with poststenotic dilatation distal to a cervical rib the morphology of the aneurysm is of proximal dilatation tapering to a normal calibre distally (Fig. 24.5). After mobilizing the subclavian artery the cervical rib should be excised, taking care not to injure the T1 nerve root which crosses the rib posteriorly. A careful search should be made for residual bands which may compress the artery. The need to remove the first rib is controversial. In patients in whom the arterial lesion is dominant there is no need to remove a normal first rib after the cervical rib has been excised completely. Some authors argue that complete decompression of this space requires removal of the first rib. After administration of heparin and application of clamps, the artery should be opened longitudinally. There is often an area of roughened tunica intima distally in the artery as a consequence of damage from a high-velocity jet of blood passing through the stenosis. This area is often about 5–10 mm in diameter and there may be adherent thrombus.

Any adherent thrombus should be removed but formal endarterectomy should not be undertaken because of the fragility of the wall. An ellipse of the wall of the artery should be excised as indicated in Figure 24.5 so that when the arteriotomy is sutured a normal calibre is restored.

A suction drain may be placed in a supraclavicular wound for 24 hours but this is not essential if there is perfect haemostasis.

Axillary artery

Proximal control of the axillary artery can be obtained through an incision through the clavipectoral fascia. The incision is made over the pectoralis major muscle 1 cm medial to the deltopectoral groove (Fig. 24.6a). The cephalic vein is preserved. The fibres of the pectoralis major are separated and the clavipectoral fascia exposed. The fascia is divided, exposing the pectoralis minor muscle. Division of this muscle gives wide exposure to the apex of the axilla. The branches of the acromiothoracic artery perforate the fascia above the pectoralis minor (Fig. 24.6b). Care should be taken to preserve the medial pectoral nerve passing through the pectoralis minor and the lateral pectoral nerve, which passes through the clavipectoral fascia above the pectoralis minor.

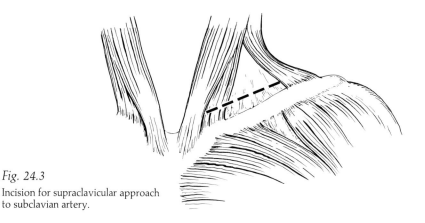

Fig. 24.3
Incision for supraclavicular approach to subclavian artery.

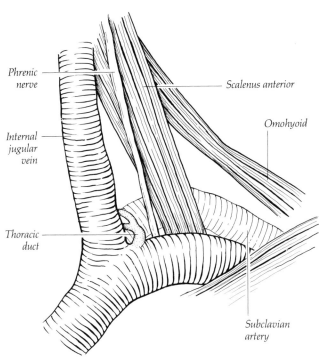

Fig. 24.4
Exposure of vessels before division of scalenus anterior.

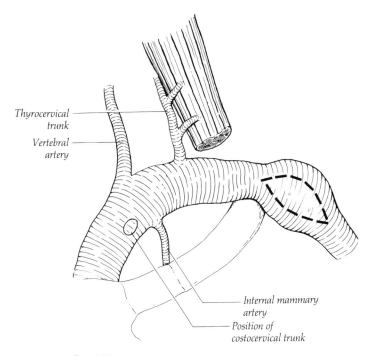

Fig. 24.5
Branches of subclavian artery and anatomy and repair of post-stenotic aneurysm.

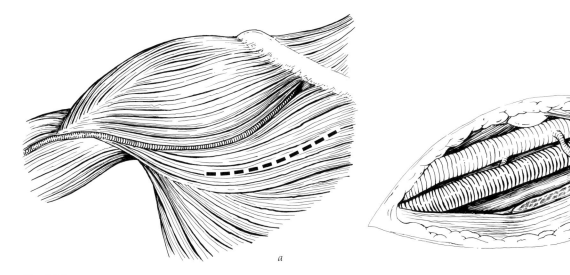

Fig. 24.6
(a) Infraclavicular approach to axillary artery—incision. (b) Detail of dissection.

The distal axillary artery is approached through a transverse incision made between the anterior and posterior axillary folds (Fig. 24.7a) as in the approach to the first rib or the axillary lymph nodes. The axillary vein lies across the anterior and inferior aspect of the artery and is the first major structure encountered. The median nerve is formed medial to the artery by the junction of its medial and lateral trunks, which pass in front of the artery (Fig. 24.7b).

It is suggested that an inlay technique be used for the repair to avoid the risk of damaging nerves and veins during attempts to excise the aneurysm. The collateral circulation at this level is very well developed, so that it will be necessary to suture from within the aneurysm several branches arising from it. The defect can be bridged using autogenous vein or prosthetic material.

Aneurysm of retro-oesophageal subclavian artery

The right subclavian artery arising as the most distal branch of the aortic arch is the commonest congenital anomaly of the arch. There have been a number of reports of aneurysm development in the part of the artery adjacent to the aorta. The lesions are commonly asymptomatic, being discovered as a mediastinal mass. Pressure on the oesophagus and trachea may occur and death from rupture has been reported.

A left lateral thoracotomy gives the best exposure of the origin of the artery which is divided between clamps and oversewn. Distally the artery is approached via a supraclavicular incision and divided. The aneurysmal segment is mobilized by careful blunt dissection and removed. Blood flow is restored to the arm by anastomosing the distal subclavian artery to the side of the right common carotid artery.

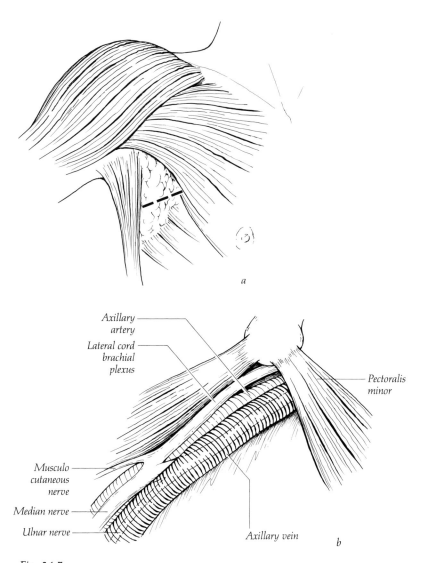

Fig. 24.7
(a) Axillary approach to axillary artery—incision. (b) Detail of dissection.

2. ULNAR ARTERY

This rare lesion is important because it may cause severe ischaemia of the fingers and is easily treated. It results from damage to the ulnar artery in the region of the hook of the hamate bone when the hypothenar region of the hand is used as a hammer ('hypothenar hammer syndrome'). The dominant hand is generally involved and in most patients there is a clear history of use of the hand which predisposes to the lesion. Histologically there is degeneration of the tunica media which presumably weakens the wall and allows the lumen to increase. Thrombus forms within the aneurysm sac and this thrombus may embolize.

CLINICAL FEATURES

Clinically there is tenderness localized to the area of the hook of the hamate bone and a pulsatile mass may be felt. Digital ischaemia characteristically affects the ring and little fingers. Compression of the superficial branch of the ulnar nerve may result in loss of sensation in these fingers.

Angiography should be performed to exclude more proximal lesions and to demonstrate the aneurysm.

OPERATION

Treatment is to excise the aneurysm. If the palmar arch is complete and there are no signs of severe ischaemia of the fingers the ulnar artery may be ligated. Figure 24.8 demonstrates the relationships between the ulnar artery and the ulnar nerve. If microsurgical skills are available a short interposition vein graft may be inserted. Preliminary thrombolytic therapy may clear thrombus from the digital arteries.

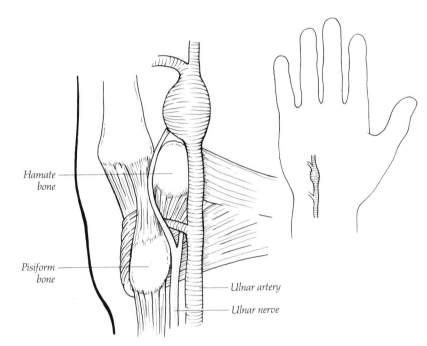

Fig. 24.8
Aneurysm of ulnar artery.

3. CAROTID ARTERY

This discussion is confined to aneurysm of the extracranial carotid arteries. These lesions are rare, and are said to represent 0.4–4% of peripheral aneurysms. They comprise 1–2% of operations on the carotid arteries. They are rarely associated with other aneurysms (in contrast to popliteal and femoral aneurysms).

In the reports in the literature, the definition of an aneurysm is often not clear. This situation has been helped by studies comparing the diameter of the common, external and internal carotid arteries (van Urk & de Jong 1990). An aneurysm of the internal carotid artery can be defined in terms of the ratio of its diameter to that of the common carotid artery. The diameter of the proximal part of the internal carotid artery (called the carotid bulb) is normally 20% greater than that of the common carotid artery. It can be considered aneurysmal if it is more than 50% greater in diameter than the common carotid artery. Using similar reasoning, the internal carotid artery beyond the carotid bulb can be considered aneurysmal if its diameter is greater than that of the common carotid artery. Aneurysms of the common and external carotid arteries are very rare.

PATHOGENESIS

The predominant cause is atherosclerosis. The aneurysm may be fusiform or saccular. Most of the lesions are in the region of the bifurcation of the common carotid artery, with the proximal internal carotid artery being the most common site. However, they may occur anywhere from the arch of the aorta to the base of the skull.

Different patterns of aneurysm are shown in Figure 24.9.

False aneurysms following trauma or surgery are a small but important group. There is a long list of other possible causes but these are great rarities.

Dissection of the wall of the carotid artery may occur spontaneously or following trauma or angiography. Spontaneous dissection is more common in younger women. These lesions cause symptoms from ischaemia due to arterial occlusion and not rupture. They are generally treated by anticoagulation and observation. Healing with recanalization is the usual result although there may be a residual neurological deficit.

CLINICAL FEATURES

Patients may present with symptoms of a mass or with cerebral ischaemia. Cerebral ischaemia is present in about 50% of cases (Zwolak et al 1984) and may be hemispheric, resulting in transient ischaemic attacks or stroke, or retinal, causing amaurosis fugax. The cause of the transient ischaemia may be embolism from the thrombus in the aneurysm or associated carotid stenosis.

In many patients the mass is asymptomatic, being discovered on routine examination. Enlargement may result in pressure symptoms. Local pain is common and the pain may be referred to the ear or head. Horner's syndrome may occur, as may palsies of the cranial nerves IX–XII.

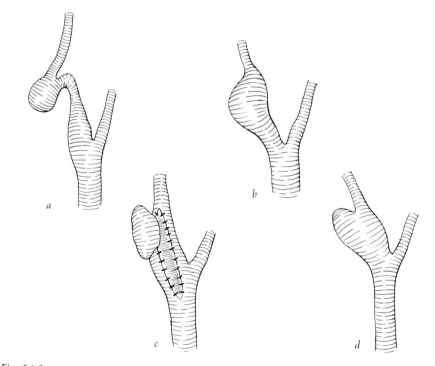

Fig. 24.9
Patterns of internal carotid aneurysm. (a) Saccular. (b) Fusiform. (c) Localized failure of suture line. (d) Postoperative with diffuse enlargement of patch.

The natural history is for the mass to enlarge slowly, although the rate of progression is unpredictable. Non-infected aneurysms rarely rupture and there is only anecdotal evidence on how often cerebral ischaemia develops. Thus conservative treatment is usually adopted for small asymptomatic atherosclerotic aneurysms. It should be noted that the evidence from small series suggests that aneurysms where there are symptoms of cerebral ischaemia are likely to be followed by stroke if not treated by operation (Zwolak et al 1984). Rapid enlargement, especially when accompanied by severe pain and/or fever, suggests a mycotic aneurysm. Rupture may occur externally to the skin or internally into the pharynx.

INVESTIGATION

It is important to distinguish aneurysm from a tortuous or kinked carotid artery. Carotid angiography is the major investigation. It will confirm that a mass is an aneurysm and demonstrate its extent. This information is essential to plan operation. Computed tomographic (CT) scanning may demonstrate the width of the aneurysm and may be the first investigation performed. Duplex ultrasound scanning may be used to monitor the progress of an aneurysm.

MANAGEMENT

Operation is advised for aneurysms of significant size which are causing symptoms due to pressure or cerebral ischaemia. Asymptomatic lesions in elderly patients may be treated conservatively and the size monitored by ultrasound scans performed at 6–12 monthly intervals. Mycotic aneurysms require surgery as soon as possible because of the risk of rupture. Patients with false aneurysms following surgery are advised to have the lesion repaired

because of the likelihood of progressive enlargement.

OPERATION

The major determinant of the operative technique is the upper level of the aneurysm. There must be sufficient distal artery available to allow the performance of an anastomosis.

Resection

The principles of operation are similar to those described for other regions, with the addition of the need to maintain cerebral perfusion.

The area of the incision may be infiltrated with saline solution containing adrenaline 1:200 000. The incision begins 1 cm inferior to the tip of the mastoid process and curves forward into an appropriate skin crease, taking care to stay well clear of the angle of the mandible in order to avoid the mandibular branch of the facial nerve (Fig. 24.10). The platysma muscle is divided. The external jugular vein is the first major structure encountered. Lying close to its posterior aspect is the greater auricular nerve, which should be mobilized and preserved.

The anterior border of the sternomastoid muscle is dissected and retracted posteriorly. This dissection normally extends from the omohyoid muscle below and cranially until the tendinous fibres of the attachment to the mastoid process can be seen.

The internal jugular vein can be seen through the deep layer of the investing cervical fascia and the carotid pulse can be felt deep to the vein. The fascia over the vein is divided and the anterior edge of the vein identified. Dissection continues along this edge throughout the length of the wound (Fig. 24.10). The major landmark is the common facial vein, which enters the anterior aspect of the internal jugular vein at the level of the hyoid bone and which overlies the carotid bifurcation. This vein should be ligated and divided. It is usually the only major tributary encountered but there may be other significant tributaries and these are more likely to be found if the common facial vein is small.

Retraction of the internal jugular vein reveals the carotid vessels. The precise dissection to be carried out depends on the anatomy of the aneurysm.

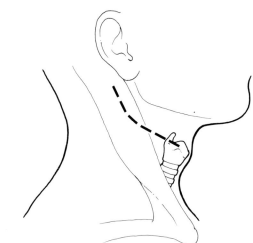

Fig. 24.10
Incision to approach internal carotid artery.

Aneurysm of proximal internal carotid artery

The dissection is the same as that carried out when performing carotid endarterectomy (Fig. 24.11). The same care must be taken to avoid dislodging embolic material from the lumen. With large or high lesions, it may be difficult to dissect the aneurysm without handling it. The nerve descendens hypoglossi may be seen on the superficial aspect of the common carotid artery. This should be preserved if possible. The common carotid artery is dissected and encircled with a tape. Care should be taken to avoid the vagus nerve, which lies posteriorly between the common carotid artery and the internal jugular vein. The common carotid artery is dissected towards the bifurcation.

The proximal part of the external carotid artery is dissected. This lies anterior and medial to the internal carotid artery and can be identified by having branches. The first of these, the superior thyroid artery, may arise close to the carotid bifurcation, so that it may not be easy to decide whether it arises from the external or common carotid artery. The external carotid artery is encircled with a tape.

Attention is now turned to the aneurysm and the internal carotid artery. The ease with which the internal carotid artery can be dissected depends on the diameter and length of the aneurysm. Dissection proceeds along the anterior aspect of the aneurysm, which may be retracted gently. The next major landmark superficial to the artery is the posterior belly of the digastric muscle. The lower border of this muscle should be dissected.

The hypoglossal nerve should be identified. This is best found by following cranially the nerve descendens hypoglossi. Dissecting along the posterior aspect of the nerve will lead to the trunk of the hypoglossal nerve as it courses forwards superficial to the carotid vessels, just inferior to the posterior belly of the digastric muscle. The hypoglossal nerve should be separated carefully from the internal carotid artery. The internal carotid artery is encircled with a tape.

Further distal exposure can be obtained by mobilizing the hypoglossal nerve more extensively. This will involve ligating and dividing the lower sternomastoid branch of the occipital artery and associated veins which tether the nerve. The posterior belly of the digastric muscle can then be dissected and divided. The glossopharyngeal nerve and the pharyngeal branch of the vagus nerve are encountered running forwards anterior to the internal carotid artery. The accessory nerve lies posterolateral to the internal carotid artery and anterior to the internal jugular vein as it passes laterally. The vagus nerve lies posterolateral to the internal carotid artery. Figure 24.12 shows the relationship between the cranial nerves and the carotid arteries. The best technique for avoiding damage to the nerves is to keep the dissection as close as possible to the artery. In this way a further length of internal carotid artery can be obtained.

The adequacy of the collateral supply to the brain should be assessed. This may be done by measuring the blood pressure in the internal carotid artery when the common and external carotid arteries are clamped. A residual pressure of greater than 50 mmHg indicates that there is adequate cerebral perfusion and it is not essential to insert a shunt to maintain cerebral perfusion. Some surgeons prefer to monitor the response of the electroencephalogram to a trial period of carotid clamping. If signs of cerebral ischaemia appear, a shunt is inserted. This may be carried out at any time while the carotid arteries are clamped. Others advocate the use of a shunt in every case because of reports of a high rate of postoperative stroke in these patients (Thompson & Talkington 1990).

Heparin 5000 units is injected intravenously and clamps applied to the three carotid arteries. If shunting is used, the shunt is inserted as soon as possible after the clamps are applied.

If the carotid arteries are tortuous it may be possible to excise the aneurysm and reanastomose the ends (Fig. 24.13a).

If this is not possible (Fig. 24.13b), an interposition graft will be necessary. Long saphenous vein is the preferred material. A segment of the vein is dissected and reversed and anastomosed to bridge the defect. If an intraluminal shunt is used to preserve cerebral perfusion (Fig. 24.14) it is possible to place the vein graft over the shunt, which is removed just before the second (usually the proximal) anastomosis is completed. It is not necessary to excise all the aneurysm and adopting this policy may reduce the chances of injuring a cranial nerve. However, the cranial nerves are most at risk during the distal part of the dissection and if it is necessary to replace the distal clamp because of bleeding from the suture line.

If the aneurysm is small and fusiform, it may be repaired by excising a longitudinal strip from the wall of the aneurysm, performing an endarterectomy if necessary, and closing the wall by direct suture (cf. Fig. 24.5). This technique may be applied to the reduction of a vein patch, which had been made too large when placed at the time of carotid endarterectomy.

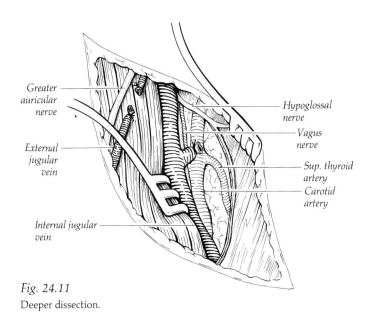

Fig. 24.11
Deeper dissection.

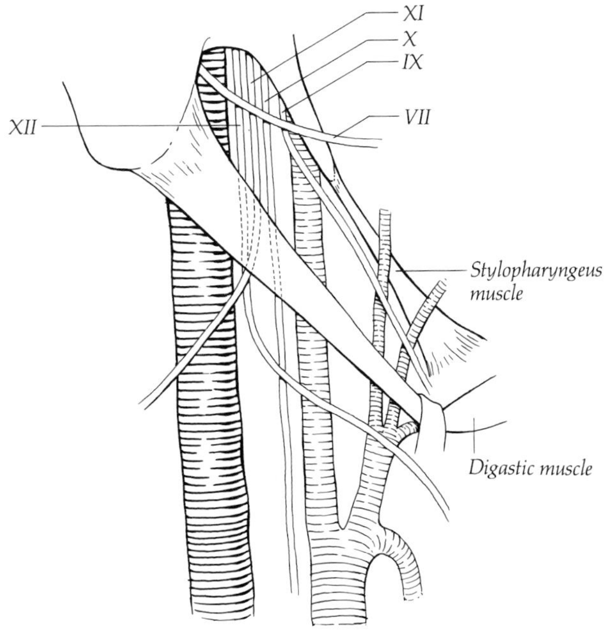

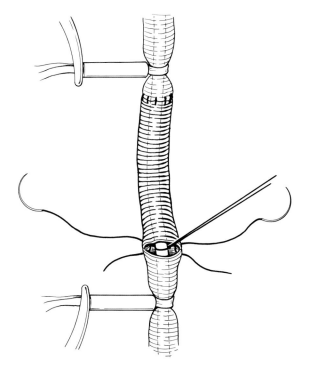

Fig. 24.12
Relationship between cranial nerves and carotid arteries.

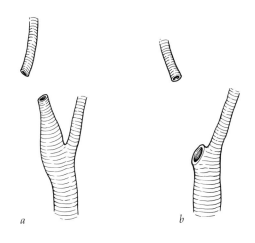

Fig. 24.13
Repair of aneurysms shown in Figure 24.9a and b, respectively.

Fig. 24.14
Vein graft sutured in presence of inlying shunt.

Before the completion of the anastomoses, great care should be taken to ensure that there is no material in the lumen which might embolize to the brain. The lumen is irrigated with heparinized saline solution and each vessel flushed by transiently releasing the clamp. A particular routine is adopted for removing the clamps. The clamps on the external and internal carotid arteries are loosened for several seconds and the clamp on the internal carotid artery is reapplied. The clamp on the common carotid artery is opened and finally the clamp on the internal carotid artery is removed. The reason for this routine is to allow any embolic material which may be in the lumen of the internal carotid artery to be flushed into the external carotid artery, where embolism is not likely to result in harmful effects.

When the suture line is dry a drain is placed to the region of the anastomoses and the wound closed.

Aneurysm of the distal internal carotid artery

These are commonly traumatic in origin due to impingement on adjacent vertebrae. There are a number of techniques for displaying the internal carotid artery up to the base of the skull. Anatomical studies (Mock et al 1991) have shown that continuation of the conventional dissection with division of the posterior belly of the digastric muscle will expose the internal carotid artery to approximately the level of the middle of the first cervical vertebra (see Fig. 24.12 for the relationships between the internal carotid artery and the cranial nerves). Anterior subluxation of the mandible increases the exposure to the upper limit of C1 and excision of the styloid process allows dissection of the internal carotid artery up to 10–12 mm from its entry to the carotid canal. Higher exposure requires a transmastoid approach.

If it is impossible to perform a carotid reconstruction in the neck, ligation of the internal carotid artery is the preferred option. This must be preceded by a test of the tolerance of the hemisphere to ischaemia because carotid ligation will be followed by stroke in 20–33% of cases. The carotid back-pressure technique is the simplest and has been described above. If the pressure is adequate the carotid artery is ligated and divided. The region of the bifurcation should be repaired carefully to avoid leaving a sump in which thrombus might form and embolize to the external carotid artery. If the pressure is inadequate a transcranial bypass should be performed. This involves anastomosing the superficial temporal artery to a parietal branch of the middle cerebral artery.

Postoperative aneurysm

Loss of the tissue planes as a consequence of the previous surgery make the dissection more difficult and increases the risk of damage to the cranial nerves. If infection is the cause there is a serious risk of haemorrhage and of compromise to the cerebral circulation during attempts to control the haemorrhage.

Non-infected false aneurysm
This may exist in two forms:

1.   Partial separation of the arteriotomy suture line (Fig. 24.9d). The bleeding is confined initially by the surrounding tissues. As the aneurysm enlarges it becomes more easily palpable. Progressive expansion is likely. There should be a careful search for the presence of infection which may present in an identical manner.
2.   Dilatation of a vein patch (Fig. 24.9d). If a vein patch is too wide progressive expansion may occur and present as a postoperative aneurysm. These are said to be more likely to thrombose than to rupture (Lord 1986).

The false aneurysm from partial separation of the suture line (Fig. 24.9c) should be repaired by dissecting the vessels so that the margins of the defect can be seen clearly and repaired using a patch of autologous vein or PTFE. The dilated vein patch should be treated by excising part of the patch so that when the defect is sutured the artery will be of an appropriate calibre.

Infected—primary

These lesions are now very rare, the commonest cause in the pre-antibiotic era being spread of infection from a peritonsillar abscess. Bacteraemia is now the most likely cause. The aneurysm is treated similarly to the more common postoperative infected false aneurysm.

Infected—secondary

The principles of management of infected false aneurysms have been described in Chapter 23. This is a very serious complication of carotid endarterectomy. It may also follow performance of carotid angiography by direct puncture but changes in radiological techniques have led to the disappearance of this cause.

The infected area must be drained adequately and dead or foreign tissue excised. This means that a prosthetic patch must be removed. If the carotid back-pressure is greater than 50 mmHg, indicating that cerebral ischaemia is unlikely following carotid ligation, ligation should be considered. The onset of stroke after this manoeuvre is unpredictable and may be delayed. Its frequency may be reduced by heparinization if the risk of haemorrhage does not preclude this therapy. If the pressure is less than 50 mmHg a very serious situation exists. It may be possible to restore blood flow to the brain by placing a vein graft between the ends of the artery.

The graft should if possible be separated from the site of the infection by placing the graft external to the sternomastoid muscle. However, as outlined previously (p. 245) a vein graft does not guarantee against further bleeding. It may be possible to perform a transcranial bypass (see above). It is necessary that blood flow is maintained in the external carotid artery for this operation to be carried out. If this is not possible, the situation is desperate. It may be possible to place a vein graft between a branch of the subclavian artery and the branch on the cerebral cortex.

Traumatic

Injuries to the carotid arteries comprise 5–7% of arterial injuries. Most of the injuries are lacerations or intimal dissection but aneurysms may follow either blunt or penetrating trauma. The principles of management are as described on page 246. An aneurysm of the internal carotid artery should be repaired using a saphenous vein interposition graft. The external carotid artery may be ligated. Aneurysm of the common carotid artery should be treated by interposition synthetic graft of approximately 8 mm diameter. The operation is conducted as described above for atherosclerotic aneurysm. When dealing with acute traumatic aneurysms it should be remembered that control of the arteries may be easier than control of the neighbouring veins from which profuse haemorrhage may occur.

RESULTS

The results from the treatment of atherosclerotic aneurysms seem to be inferior to those following carotid endarterectomy. The mortality following surgery has been reported to be 0–13%, the number of strokes 0–17%. Morbidity may also result from damage to a cranial nerve which occurs in approximately 20% of patients.

REFERENCES

Lord R S A 1986 Surgery of occlusive cerebrovascular disease. C V Mosby, St Louis, p 265
Mock C N, Lilly M P, McRae R G, Carney W I 1991 Selection of the approach to the distal internal carotid artery from the second cervical vertebra to the base of the skull. Journal of Vascular Surgery 13: 846–853
Neumayer L A, Bull D A, Hunter G C et al 1992 Atherosclerotic aneurysms of the axillary artery. Journal of Cardiovascular Surgery 33: 172–177
Thompson J E, Talkington C M 1990 The surgery of carotid aneurysms. In: Greenhalgh R M, Mannick J A, Powell J T (eds) The cause and management of aneurysms. W B Saunders, London, pp 237–244
van Urk H, de Jong K P 1990 The dimensions of the carotid bifurcation and definition of carotid artery aneurysm. In Greenhalgh R M, Mannick J A, Powell J T (eds) The cause and management of aneurysms. W B Saunders, London, pp 123–128
Zwolak R M, Whitehouse W M, Knake J E et al 1984 Atherosclerotic extracranial carotid artery aneurysms. Journal of Vascular Surgery 1: 415–422

Chapter 25

Aneurysm of branches of the abdominal aorta

RENAL ARTERY

Aneurysms of the renal arteries may occur in subjects over a wide range of age and are the commonest arterial aneurysms occurring in children. They represent about 1% of all aneurysms and 20% of visceral aneurysms. The number of cases diagnosed seems to be increasing with the wider use of angiography.

PATHOLOGY

The aetiology is uncertain in many cases but some may be congenital in origin. This is suggested by their occurrence in children and the tendency for these aneurysms to occur at bifurcations where the elastic laminae may be thinner. This is analogous to the pathology of intracranial aneurysms. Hypertension may be the precipitating factor for the growth of an aneurysm. Other causes include fibromuscular dysplasia, polyarteritis nodosa, neurofibromatosis and, in the older population, atherosclerosis. Thinning of the wall associated with fibromuscular dysplasia may lead to aneurysm formation. The frequency with which fibromuscular dysplasia is treated by balloon angioplasty might predispose to aneurysm formation but such an association does not seem to have been described. The haemodynamic changes associated with pregnancy are probably the causes of aneurysm rupture during pregnancy (Cohen & Shamash 1987). Sporadic cases have been reported following renal transplantation. These seem to arise from an anastomosis and are probably false aneurysms arising at the suture line. An arteriovenous fistula may develop following renal biopsy or percutaneous nephrolithotomy. This usually results in destruction of renal tissue and requires nephrectomy

although transarterial catheter techniques to control the fistula may be applicable.

The most common site is in the main renal artery or its first-order branches. Aneurysms may be bilateral in 20% of cases (Martin et al 1989). There is a marked female preponderance in subjects aged less than 40 years.

The precise incidence of rupture is difficult to determine although it is estimated at about 5%. However, the mortality of rupture is high (estimated at 80%). The factors which predispose to rupture are said to include pregnancy, hypertension, lack of calcification and diameter > 1.5 cm. The aneurysm is on the left side in 90% of cases where rupture occurs during pregnancy.

CLINICAL FEATURES

The aneurysms may be discovered by chance during investigation for some unrelated disorder. Angiography for the investigation of hypertension is the commonest mode of diagnosis. Unruptured aneurysms may be associated with vague upper abdominal or flank pain. Rupture is associated with severe pain in the back and loin and signs of hypovolaemia. Contained rupture is common and may be associated with anaemia rather than hypovolaemia. Haematuria may be noted. Hypertension is present in most cases. This may be renin dependent despite the absence of demonstrable renal artery stenosis in some cases. Repair of the aneurysm may result in cure of the hypertension. There may be no physical signs of unruptured aneurysms but when the aneurysm ruptures there will be upper abdominal and loin tenderness and a mass may be felt.

INDICATIONS FOR OPERATION

Aneurysms in women of child-bearing age should be repaired if further pregnancies are desired. If an aneurysm is diagnosed during pregnancy, it should be repaired forthwith because the risks of maternal and/or fetal death are greater following rupture than would be expected following elective surgery.

The indications for elective operation in other patients remain controversial. Aneurysms associated with renin production and hypertension should be repaired. Aneurysms of small size in normotensive patients can be treated conservatively (Tham et al 1985) and seem to have a benign natural history. Some advise repair of aneurysms > 1.5 cm diameter and non-calcified aneurysms are believed by some authors to be at greater risk of rupture. If there are symptoms which are attributable to expansion of the aneurysm or if the aneurysm ruptures, operation should be undertaken.

OPERATION

Elective operation
The approach will be determined by the angiographic findings. Lesions close to the aorta may be approached anteriorly as described on page 156. More distal lesions of the main artery will be approached after reflecting the colon (and duodenum on the right side). If autotransplantation is to be performed, a loin incision will be used. A variety of procedures may be carried out:

1. Aortorenal bypass grafting may be performed if the proximal part of the renal artery cannot be repaired (Fig. 25.1).
2. Solitary aneurysms at the bifurcation of the renal artery are excised (Fig. 25.2).
3. Ex vivo repair is undertaken for

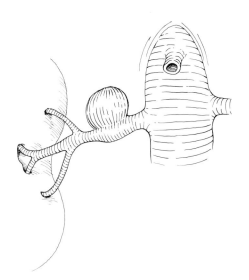

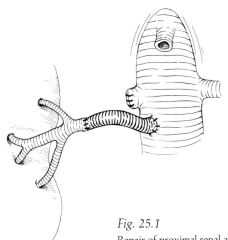

Fig. 25.1
Repair of proximal renal artery aneurysm with vein graft.

complicated multiple or distal lesions. Preoperative angiography should assess the suitability of the internal iliac artery as a graft. The operation is conducted as for a living donor nephrectomy. The important principles are to ensure adequate hydration, avoid hypotension and give mannitol (see p. 19). The renal artery and vein are divided and the ureter mobilized or divided. The kidney is flushed with renal preservation solution and packed in ice slush.

The repair is carried out using microsurgical techniques. Figure 25.3 shows an aneurysm within the hilum of the kidney with three segmental branches coming from it. An interposition vein graft has been used and the remaining branches will be anastomosed to the side of this graft. The graft may be a segment of long saphenous vein or the internal iliac artery. The kidney is reimplanted into the opposite iliac fossa with the arterial anastomosis to the external or internal iliac artery and the venous anastomosis to the external iliac vein. The operation is facilitated if one team performs the nephrectomy and prepares for the reimplantation while a second team performs the repair.

4. Nephrectomy is occasionally necessary if the lesions are beyond repair.

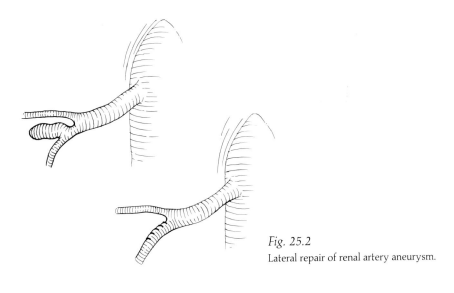

Fig. 25.2
Lateral repair of renal artery aneurysm.

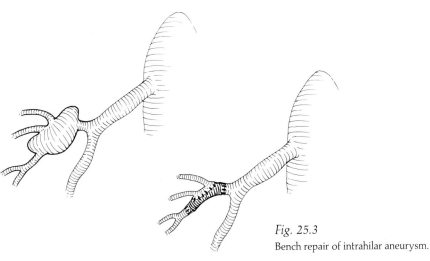

Fig. 25.3
Bench repair of intrahilar aneurysm.

Emergency repair

Laparotomy is undertaken for intra-abdominal bleeding of undetermined cause so that wide exposure is necessary. A long midline incision is preferred. The diagnosis is made on finding retroperitoneal haemorrhage on one side of the aorta. The aorta is dissected below the left renal vein, which is mobilized as described on page 156. Dissection continues upwards until the origin of the renal artery is found. This is dissected and clamped.

The renal artery is dissected towards the hilum of the kidney. In rare cases it is possible to identify the renal artery distal to the aneurysm and place an interposition graft. However, almost always the disruption of the hilar region, the distal location of the aneurysm and the shocked state of the patient require that nephrectomy be undertaken. It is essential to check that the patient has a contralateral kidney before undertaking nephrectomy.

REFERENCES

Cohen J R, Shamash F S 1987 Ruptured renal artery aneurysms during pregnancy. Journal of Vascular Surgery 6: 51–59

Martin R S, Meacham P W, Ditesheim J A, Mulherin J L, Edwards W H 1989 Renal artery aneurysm: selective treatment for hypertension and prevention of rupture. Journal of Vascular Surgery 9: 26–34

Tham G, Ekelund L, Herrlin K, Lindstedt E L, Olin T, Bergentz S-E 1983 Renal artery aneurysms. Annals of Surgery 197: 348–352

Chapter 26

Splanchnic artery aneurysms

Introduction

These may occur on the main branches from the aorta or on the smaller branches of these arteries. The table (derived from Stanley & Zelenock 1989) gives the relative frequency of these aneurysms.

Celiac trunk	4 %
Splenic artery	60 %
Hepatic artery	20 %
Gastroduodenal artery	1.5%
Pancreatico-duodenal/pancreatic	2 %
Superior mesenteric artery	5.5%
Jejunal/ileal/colic branches	3 %
Left gastric/epiploic artery	4 %

1. SPLENIC ARTERY

The splenic artery is the commonest site of visceral aneurysms, comprising about 60% of the total. They occur more commonly in women and are associated with pregnancy and multiparity and, although the natural history is well known, surgical treatment remains controversial.

AETIOLOGY

The changes in the wall of the artery described below which are associated with pregnancy are almost certainly important. Evidence of atherosclerosis at other sites is unusual. They may be more common in patients with portal hypertension. Pancreatitis is an important aetiological factor in the development of false aneurysms. The activated pancreatic enzymes damage the wall of the artery and cause aneurysms to develop.

PATHOLOGY

The commonest location is at the distal branching of the artery and multiple splenic aneurysms may be found in 20% of cases. Histological evidence of atherosclerosis is present in almost all cases (Trastek et al 1985); however, the age and sex distribution and the association with pregnancy suggest another cause. Histological changes in the artery wall associated with pregnancy include intimal hyperplasia and fragmentation of elastic laminae. It is suggested that these changes weaken the wall and the haemodynamic changes associated with pregnancy result in aneurysm formation, and the atheromatous changes are secondary. The aneurysms occur most commonly in the distal part of the artery and are multiple in 10–30% of cases.

CLINICAL FEATURES

Female patients outnumber males by 5:1 (see Trastek et al 1985 for review). The majority (about 80%) are asymptomatic when the aneurysm is detected. Some patients will have non-specific abdominal pain. There are no characteristic physical signs. A mass may be palpable in 3% of patients.

About 5% of patients present with rupture, the features of which are severe upper abdominal pain and hypovolaemia. The aneurysm may rupture into the peritoneal cavity or into an adjacent viscus such as the stomach or the pancreatic duct, when it presents as gastrointestinal haemorrhage. In pregnant patients a ruptured visceral aneurysm is four times more likely to be of the splenic artery than of the renal artery, which is the next most common site. The condition may mimic other causes of circulatory collapse in pregnancy, such as placental separation, uterine rupture and amniotic fluid embolism.

INVESTIGATION

The aneurysm is often identified from the finding of a calcified left upper quadrant mass on plain radiographs of the abdomen. Computed tomographic (CT) scanning may make the diagnosis but, if necessary, the diagnosis can be confirmed by angiography.

INDICATIONS FOR OPERATION

The natural history of these aneurysms suggests that operation should be undertaken when this lesion is detected in a woman who is or who may become pregnant. As more of these cases are diagnosed the percentage which rupture decreases and in some series is less than 5%. Certainly the incidence of rupture is very low in patients who have been treated conservatively and the mortality following rupture in non-pregnant patients is also less than 10%. These figures argue for a conservative approach to surgery. Rupture during pregnancy is most common in the third trimester and is associated with high maternal (about 70%) and fetal (about 90%) mortality.

Operation should be undertaken if symptoms can reasonably be attributed to the aneurysm or if rupture occurs.

Occlusion of the splenic artery by emboli or coils introduced into the artery may be undertaken. However, it is essential to ensure that the artery distal to the aneurysm is occluded in addition to the inflow artery.

OPERATION

Aneurysm of the splenic artery may be approached via a left subcostal or epigastric midline incision. The lesser sac is opened by dividing the gastrocolic omentum and short gastric arteries (Fig. 26.1a). The superior border of the pancreas is displayed after retracting the stomach cranially and the transverse colon caudally.

The procedure to be carried out depends on the location of the aneurysm:

1.   Aneurysms in the hilum of the spleen (Fig. 26.1b) may not be able to be controlled proximally and distally without resection of the spleen. If resection is necessary, the patient should be warned of the possibility of overwhelming postsplenectomy sepsis and immunized against pneumococcal infection.
2.   If a ligature can be placed on the artery distal to the aneurysm, the spleen should be preserved. The aneurysm is treated by excision of the aneurysm and ligation of the inflow and outflow

arteries. This should include branches running from the aneurysm to the pancreas. There is evidence that phagocytic function of the spleen is preserved after this procedure.

When a hilar aneurysm has ruptured, splenectomy will be required if the bleeding is profuse. This is carried out in the usual way for dealing with a ruptured spleen. The lienorenal ligament is divided and the spleen displaced anteriorly until clamps can be applied to the hilum. On rare occasions it may be seen that the aneurysm is clearly proximal to the hilum and it may be possible to control the bleeding without removing the spleen.

Bleeding from the splenic artery associated with pancreatitis may be retroperitoneal or intragastric. In these cases suture ligation of the bleeding artery is carried out.

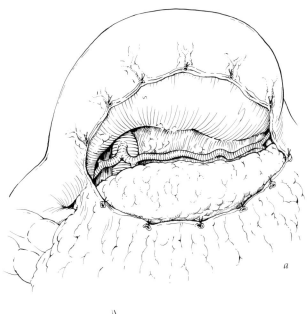

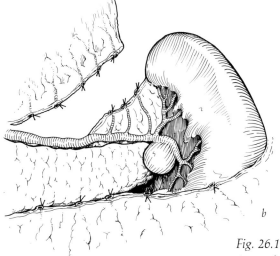

Fig. 26.1
Approach to proximal and distal splenic artery.

2. HEPATIC ARTERY

Aneurysms of the hepatic artery are the second commonest of the aneurysms of the visceral vessels, being involved in 20% of these cases.

AETIOLOGY

The commonest cause of these lesions is degenerative, although intrinsic disease of the arterial wall from Ehlers–Danlos syndrome or polyarteritis nodosa may occur. Mycotic aneurysms are relatively common (cf. aneurysms of the superior mesenteric artery). Aneurysm formation may follow liver biopsy or blunt or penetrating abdominal trauma.

PATHOLOGY

The major cause is said to be degeneration of the tunica media. True aneurysms tend to be saccular. The aneurysm arises from the common hepatic artery or the right hepatic artery in 90% of cases.

CLINICAL FEATURES

These lesions are more common in men, in contrast to aneurysms of the splenic artery. They may present without symptoms but rupture is the presenting feature in 40–50%. Symptoms tend to be non-specific but pressure on bile ducts may cause jaundice or the symptoms may mimic cholecystitis or pancreatitis. Expansion of the aneurysm may produce biliary pain. Intrahepatic rupture occurs in 50% of cases. The features are of gastrointestinal bleeding, abdominal pain and jaundice.

INVESTIGATION

These aneurysms may present as a calcified mass in the right upper quadrant and may need to be differentiated from gallstone or hydatid cyst. They may be diagnosed on ultrasound or computed tomographic (CT) scanning of the liver. There may be biochemical evidence of obstruction to the bile duct. Angiography is likely to be necessary to determine the exact site of origin of the aneurysm. Primary aneurysms arise from the main trunk of the artery or, occasionally, from its major branches.

OPERATION

Operation should be advised once the diagnosis has been made because of the risk of rupture.

The treatment required depends on the location of the aneurysm:

1. For intrahepatic lesions, catheter techniques should be used to occlude the branch(es) of the hepatic artery feeding the aneurysm. These techniques are particularly effective in dealing with cases of haematobilia.
2. For extrahepatic lesions, resection and repair should be undertaken. If the lesion is proximal to the gastroduodenal artery, proximal and distal ligation has been employed safely.

A midline incision should be used. The region of the coeliac axis should be approached above the stomach through the lesser omentum. This approach (see p. 144) allows clamping of the aorta, should this be necessary in cases of rupture. In elective cases the coeliac axis and its branches are dissected at the aorta between the crura of the diaphragm. The hepatic artery is identified and taped (Fig. 26.2).

The distal part of the hepatic artery should be dissected in the free edge of the lesser omentum (Fig. 26.3). Care

must be taken not to damage the bile duct during this dissection. The major uncontrolled branch remains the gastroduodenal artery. This runs between the first part of the duodenum and the neck of the pancreas and lies immediately to the right of the peritoneal reflection at the right side of the lesser sac of the peritoneum. The illustration shows an aneurysm arising close to the origin of the gastroduodenal artery. In this case it may be difficult to dissect the artery separately from the aneurysm. When the aneurysm is opened profuse back-bleeding can be controlled by sutures placed within the aneurysm.

When the vessels are controlled, heparin is given and clamps are applied to the arteries. The aneurysm is opened and intraluminal thrombus and debris removed. Small arteries back-bleeding into the aneurysm may need to be controlled.

Reconstruction should be completed by interposing a saphenous vein graft between the ends of the artery.

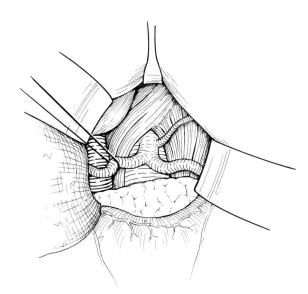

Fig. 26.2
Approach to origin of hepatic artery.

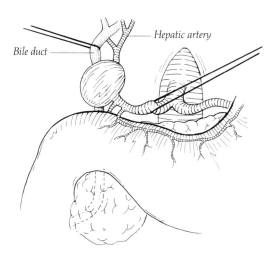

Fig. 26.3
Dissection of distal hepatic artery.

3. SUPERIOR MESENTERIC ARTERY

Aneurysms of the superior mesenteric artery and its branches are rare, comprising fewer than 10% of peripheral aneurysms. They are probably being recognized more frequently because of the widespread availability of angiography. Of particular importance is the observation that the commonest group are mycotic aneurysms, which account for more than half of the cases. The source of infection is commonly bacteraemia from intravenous drug use or bacterial endocarditis. Infection may occur by spread from adjacent organs. Gram-positive organisms, especially *Staphylococcus aureus* and *Streptococcus* species are the most common bacteria found. However, no organisms can be isolated in about 25% of cases presumed to be mycotic in origin. True aneurysms may occur in association with fibromuscular dysplasia, atherosclerosis or Ehlers–Danlos syndrome. False aneurysms may follow blunt or penetrating trauma.

CLINICAL FEATURES

There are no specific clinical features to assist in making the diagnosis. There may be a variety of upper abdominal symptoms. A mass will only be felt if the aneurysm is large.

INVESTIGATION

Computed tomographic (CT) scanning is the most helpful method of diagnosis. There is seldom enough calcification in the wall to show on plain radiographs of the abdomen. Angiography should be performed to define the anatomy prior to surgery.

These aneurysms are said to have a high propensity to rupture. This may occur into the peritoneal cavity or into the lumen of the bowel, this being one of the rarer causes of arterioenteric fistula.

OPERATION

A long midline incision should be performed. The aneurysm will be palpable in the base of the mesentery. The approach to be taken depends on whether the aneurysm is ruptured and how far distal it is in the superior mesenteric artery. If the aneurysm is ruptured the first step in the procedure should be to prepare to clamp the supracoeliac aorta (see p. 144).

If it is not necessary to clamp the aorta the origin of the superior mesenteric artery can be approached. This is best achieved by dissecting the anterior aspect of the aorta, starting below and finishing above the left renal vein. The trunk of the superior mesenteric artery lies in the root of the mesentery and is just anterior to the area of dissection (Fig. 26.4). Continuing the dissection of the anterior wall of the aorta will lead to the acute angle made by the origin of the superior mesenteric artery from the aorta (Fig. 26.5). The left renal vein lies within this angle. The aim of the dissection is to display both sides of the origin of the superior mesenteric artery to allow the application of a curved clamp to the aorta, thus controlling the superior mesenteric artery.

The trunk of the superior mesenteric artery can be approached directly in the left edge of the root of the mesentery. The area for beginning this dissection is indicated in Figure 26.4. The dissection is usually straightforward because the corresponding veins are on the right side of the artery. It may be necessary to mobilize the duodenojejunal flexure to gain access to this area.

Attention is then turned to gaining distal control of the artery. If the aneurysm only involves the proximal part of the artery, this is best approached through the left posterolateral aspect of the root of the mesentery as described.

If this approach is not suitable the superior mesenteric artery is approached from the anterior aspect of the mesentery. The small bowel is retracted inferiorly and the artery sought by dissection in the base of the transverse mesocolon. The artery may have decreased substantially in calibre by the time it crosses the duodenum after giving off a number of jejunal branches. There are a number of veins accompanying the arteries and they may make dissection difficult.

After administration of heparin, clamps are applied. The aneurysm is incised, the contents are removed and sent for bacteriological examination and culture. If it is believed that the aneurysm is infected as much as possible of the wall of the aneurysm should be removed.

An alternative approach is to use a midline or left thoracoabdominal approach as described on page 101 for the retroperitoneal exposure of the aorta. This approach may be preferred if

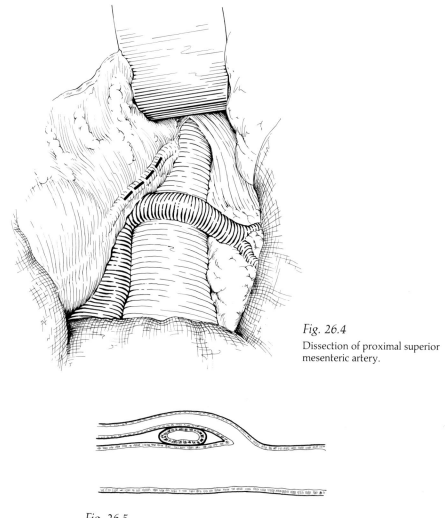

Fig. 26.4
Dissection of proximal superior mesenteric artery.

Fig. 26.5
Relationships of aorta, left renal vein and superior mesenteric artery.

complete exposure of the aorta and its branches is required, as in cases of penetrating injury where there may not be complete information about the extent of the injury.

Reconstruction

If the aneurysm extends proximal to the first jejunal branch, ischaemia is likely to follow ligation, so that arterial reconstruction should be performed.

The preferred method of reconstruction is to oversew the proximal end of the superior mesenteric artery and place a bypass graft of saphenous vein between the infrarenal aorta and the distal end of the superior mesenteric artery (Fig 26.6).

It is sometimes possible to perform the repair using the inlay technique. Prosthetic materials may be used if there is no infection.

If the aneurysm is suspected of being mycotic in origin antibiotic therapy should be continued for 6 weeks following surgery.

In some cases the aneurysm adheres to and forms a fistula into the duodenum or jejunum. In these cases the defect in the bowel will require repair as in cases of aortoenteric fistula (see p. 228).

4. COELIAC ARTERY

These aneurysms are also very rare and are most commonly degenerative in origin. Epigastric discomfort and tenderness are the commonest clinical features. A mass may be felt in about one-third of cases. Expansion or rupture of an aneurysm may produce features hard to distinguish from acute pancreatitis. The risk of rupture is estimated to be 13% (Graham et al 1985). Computed tomographic scanning is the most useful test for making the diagnosis and angiography will be necessary before planned surgery.

Surgery should be undertaken for these lesions. A left retroperitoneal approach to the coeliac artery is employed (see p. 110). If difficulty is encountered the incision should be continued into the chest through the seventh intercostal space. It will usually be necessary to clamp the aorta and oversew the origin of the coeliac axis. A graft can be placed between the distal coeliac artery and the aorta as shown in Figure 32.3 in the case of the superior mesenteric artery.

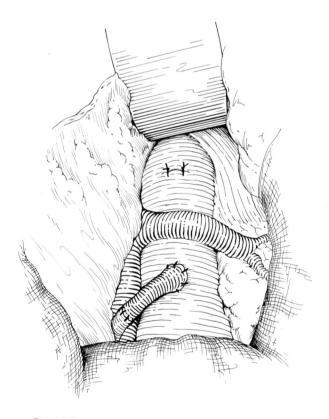

Fig. 26.6
Vein graft between infrarenal aorta and superior mesenteric artery.

5. BRANCHES OF VISCERAL ARTERIES

Aneurysms may develop on the peripheral branches of the arteries to the gut. These include the gastric and epiploic branches of the left gastric artery, the pancreaticoduodenal branches of the hepatic artery and the jejunal, ilieal and colic branches of the superior mesenteric artery. Degenerative changes in the wall of the artery is the commonest cause. Other causes include local inflammation as in pancreatitis or systemic disease, for example periarteritis nodosa and other collagen vascular disorders, bacterial endocarditis and hairy-cell leukaemia.

Clinical features range from an incidental finding during investigation of unrelated symptoms to severe haemorrhage. Aneurysms close to the wall of the intestine may produce gastrointestinal haemorrhage. If rupture does not occur into the gut, intra- or retroperitoneal haemorrhage will result. Rupture of one of these aneurysms is an important cause of spontaneous retroperitoneal haemorrhage ('abdominal apoplexy'). Pressure on local structures may produce symptoms and there have been several reports of cure of recurrent pancreatitis following resection of an aneurysm of the pancreaticoduodenal artery. Presumably the aneurysm had been pressing on the pancreatic duct.

These aneurysms should be excised when detected because the mortality following rupture approaches 50%.

Operation involves exposing the site of the aneurysm and suture ligating the vessel. Larger aneurysms may be excised for histological examination. When rupture occurs it is not usually possible to identify an aneurysm as the cause in the haemorrhagic mass that is encountered. In these cases the site of bleeding is oversewn. Ligation of these peripheral arteries does not cause distal ischaemia so that reconstruction is unnecessary.

REFERENCES

Graham L M, Stanley J C, Whitehouse W M et al 1985 Celiac artery aneurysms: historic (1745–1949) versus contemporary (1950–1984) differences in aetiology and clinical importance. Journal of Vascular Surgery 2: 757–764
Stanley J C, Zelenock G B 1989 Splanchnic artery aneurysms. In: Rutherford R B (ed) Vascular surgery. W B Saunders, Philadelphia, pp 969–983
Lal R J, Strohl J A, Piazza S, Aslam M, Ball D, Patel K 1989 Hepatic artery aneurysm. Journal of Cardiovascular Surgery 30: 509–513
Trastek V F, Pairolero P C, Bernatz P E 1985 Splenic artery aneurysms. World Journal of Surgery 9: 378–383